Preface

I should like to thank Professor Daniel Catovsky, Dr Carol Barton, Dr Helen Dodsworth, Dr Sue Fairhead, Dr Carol Hughes, Mrs Jean Mellor and Dr Marjorie Walker for help with photographs; Professor David Linch for permission to reproduce Figures 80A and 92 which are taken from *Colour guide, haematology*; and Professor Harry Smith for permission to reproduce Figures 106 and 107 which are taken from *Diagnosis in paediatric haematology*. I am grateful to the Audio-Visual Department of the Imperial College School of Medicine at St Mary's Hospital for photographing laboratory tests and for permission to publish the following Figures: 1A, 33A and B, 40B, 43A, 48, 55A and B, 63, 82, 84, 86, 88A, 96A and B, 97A and B, 98 and 101. In particular, I should like to thank the patients who gave permission for their photographs to be published in the hope that this would contribute to the education of medical students and the further education of medical graduates.

London
1997

B.J.B

Contents

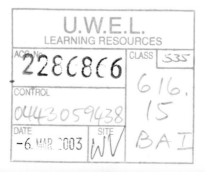

Questions

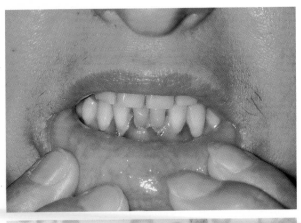

A

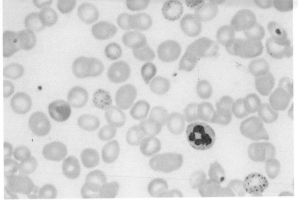

B

1. This Indian woman complained of constipation. Her blood film is shown in (B). Her haemoglobin concentration was 8.3 g/dl, the mean red cell volume (MCV) was 84.8 fl and the reticulocyte count was increased to 281 × 10⁹/L (9.4%).

a. What abnormality is shown by the blood film?
b. What abnormality is seen in the mouth?
c. What is the diagnosis?

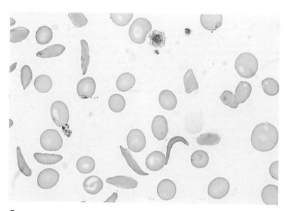

2. This blood film is from a 20-year-old African patient with recurrent limb pains, a haemoglobin concentration of 7.3 g/dl and an MCV of 93 fl.

a. What is the most significant abnormality shown?
b. What is the most likely diagnosis?
c. What test should be performed and what results would you expect?
d. Comment on the size of the platelets and given an explanation.

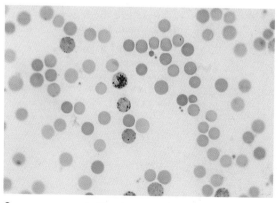

3. This is reticulocyte preparation (obtained by incubating blood with new methylene blue).

a How many reticulocytes are present?
b. Is the reticulocyte count reduced, normal or increased?

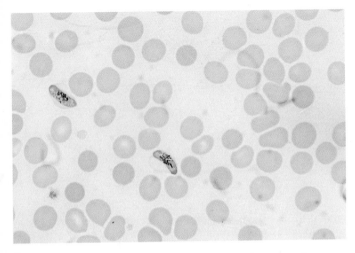

4. This blood film is of a febrile patient who recently returned from Africa.

a. What is the most significant abnormality?
b. What is the diagnosis?

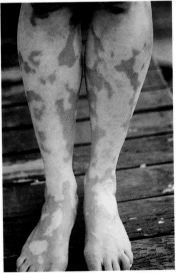

5. These are the legs of a middle-aged woman.

a. What is the diagnosis?
b. What haematological condition shows an increased incidence in patients with this abnormality of the skin?

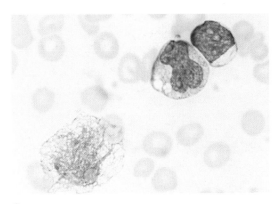

6. This is the blood film of a young man with fever, slight hepatosplenomegaly, leucocytosis, anaemia and thrombocytopenia.

a. What abnormality is shown by the smaller cell?
b. What is the likely diagnosis?

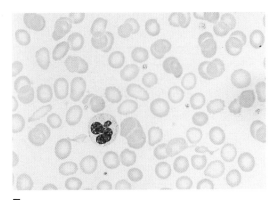

7. This is the blood film of a 60-year-old man with constipation. His diet was normal and there was no history of any preceding illness. The haemoglobin concentration was 8.2 g/dl, the MCV was 71 fl and the mean cell haemoglobin concentration (MCHC) was 27.8 g/dl.

a. What abnormalities are shown by the blood count?
b. List the two most significant abnormalities shown by the blood film.
c. What is the most likely diagnosis?
d. What test or tests would you request to confirm this diagnosis?
e. What other investigations would be important in this patient?

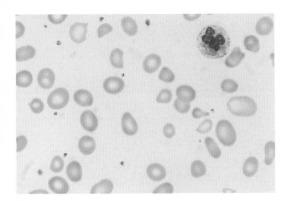

8. This is the blood film of an elderly woman who complained of lethargy, weight loss, loss of appetite and numbness of the feet. Her diet was usually good but in the preceding few weeks it had been poor as she had become anorexic. Her haemoglobin was found to be 4.5 g/dl and her MCV was 115 fl.

a. List four abnormalities shown by the blood film.
b. Which abnormalities are the most significant from the point of view of diagnosis?
c. What is the most likely diagnosis?

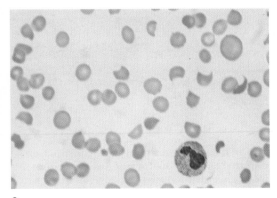

9. This is the blood film of an 8-year-old boy with oliguria, a creatinine concentration of 213 μm/L and a haemoglobin concentration of 6.5 g/dl.

a. List the four most significant abnormalities shown.
b. What is the likely nature of the anaemia?
c. What is the most likely diagnosis?

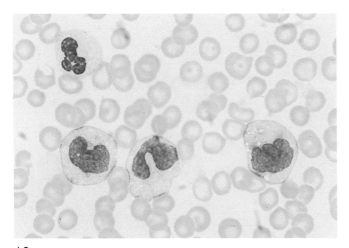

10. This is the blood film of an elderly man with mild splenomegaly and chronic anaemia, leucocytosis and thrombocytopenia.

a. Identify the four white cells shown.
b. What is the most likely diagnosis?

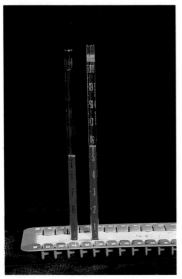

11. The photograph shows the measurement of the haematocrit or packed cell volume in two patients.

a. What is the haematocrit in each patient?
b. What is the white band at the top of the red cell column?

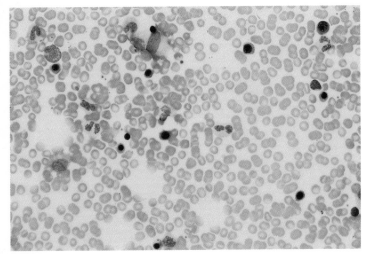

A

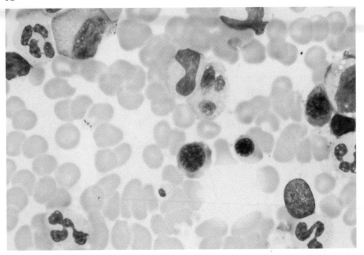

B

12. These slides show medium and high power views (A, B) of normal bone marrow, and medium and high power views (C, D: opposite) of bone marrow from a patient with a macrocytic anaemia.

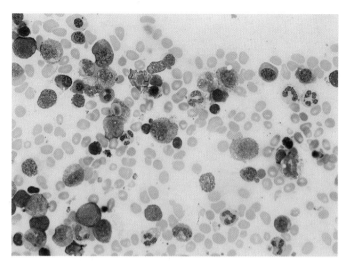

C

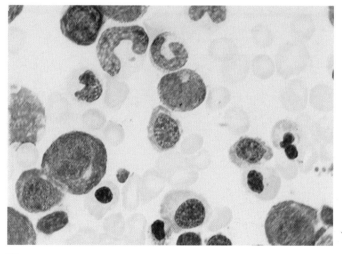

D

a. What abnormalities are shown in the patient's bone marrow (C, D)?
b. What is the diagnosis?
c. What two blood tests would be indicated in the initial investigation?

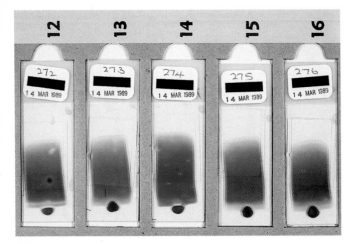

13. This is the macroscopic appearance of blood films from five patients.

a. What abnormality is shown by the central blood film?
b. What is the likely diagnosis?

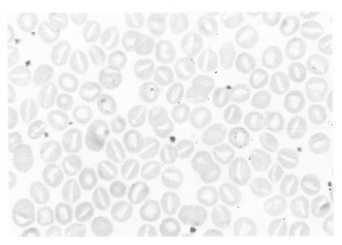

14. This is the blood film of an anaemic patient.

What two abnormalities are shown?

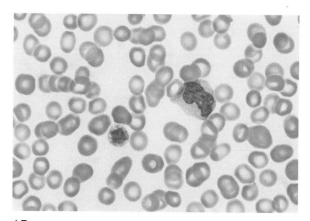

15. **This is the blood film of a patient with renal insufficiency and sensorineural deafness.**

a. What are the two most significant abnormalities in the blood film?
b. What is the most likely diagnosis?

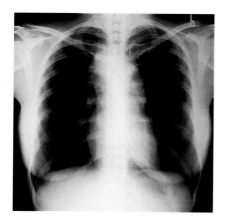

16. **This is a chest X-ray of a young woman of northern European origin who had recently noted the presence of a firm, non-tender supraclavicular lymph node. She was afebrile and no abnormality was detected on examination of the pharynx.**

a. What abnormality is present?
b. What is the most likely diagnosis?

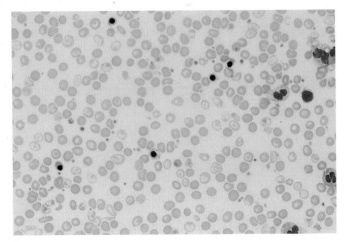

A

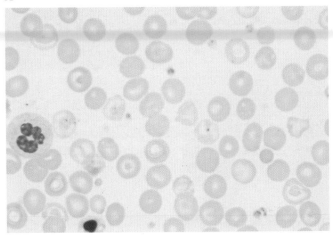

B

17. These are medium (A) and high power (B) views of the blood film of a young Cypriot woman who required regular blood transfusions from early infancy and who underwent a splenectomy.

a. List the abnormalities shown.
b. What is the most likely diagnosis?

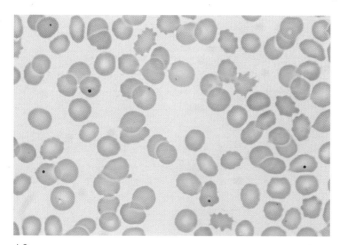

18. **This is the blood film of a patient with a previous diagnosis of autoimmune thrombocytopenic purpura.**

a. List all the abnormalities shown and offer an interpretation.
b. Discuss the treatment that this patient has received and its efficacy.

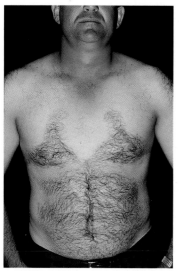

19. **This is the trunk of a patient recently treated for a haematological malignancy.**

a. What treatment has been given?
b. What is the most likely diagnosis?

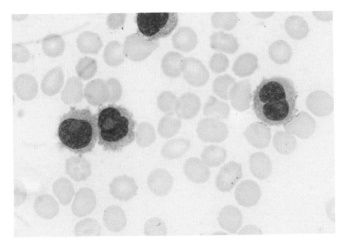

A

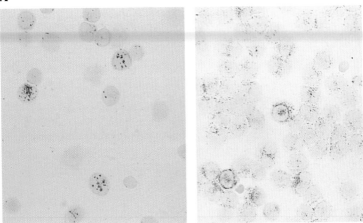

B

20. (A) Shows cells in the blood of a middle-aged man with anaemia, neutropenia, monocytopenia and thrombocytopenia. (B) shows a cytochemical reaction, acid phosphatase (left) and tartrate-resistant acid phosphatase (right).

What is the diagnosis?

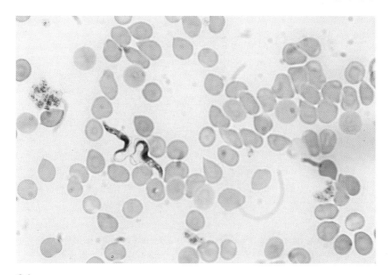

21. This is a blood film of a patient from West Africa.

a. What abnormality is shown?
b. What disease would be expected?

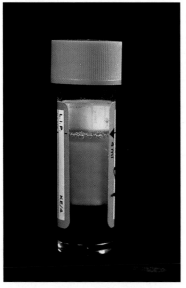

22. This is an anticoagulated blood sample from an elderly man with pallor and marked splenomegaly but with no lymphadenopathy. The blood has been allowed to sediment for several hours.

a. What two abnormalities are shown?
b. What is the most likely diagnosis?

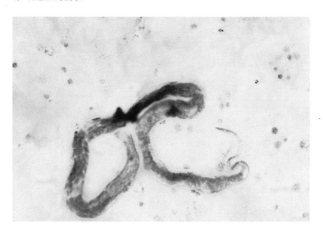

23. **This thick film was performed for the detection of malaria in a west African patient.**

The patient is infected by two types of parasite. What are they?

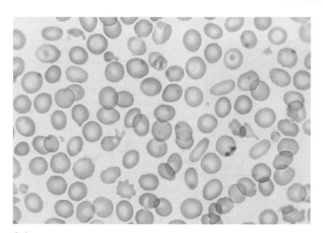

24. **This blood film is from a middle-aged Italian woman with a normal haemoglobin concentration, a high red cell count (RBC) and a reduced mean red cell volume (MCV).**

a. What abnormalities are seen?
b. What is the most likely diagnosis?
c. What test would you request to confirm the diagnosis?

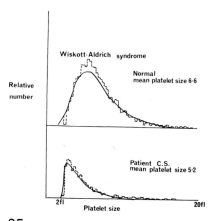

Wiskott-Aldrich syndrome

Normal
mean platelet size 6·6

Relative
number

Patient C.S.
mean platelet size 5·2

2fl   20fl
Platelet size

25. This is a histogram of platelet size performed on a Coulter Counter in a patient with Wiskott–Aldrich syndrome.

What are the features of this syndrome?

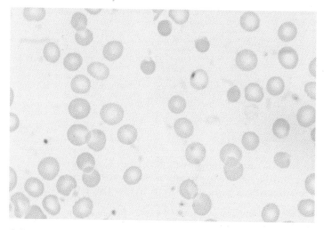

26. This blood film is from a West Indian child who developed lethargy and pallor after suffering a urinary tract infection.

a. What abnormality is present?
b. What diagnosis is most likely?

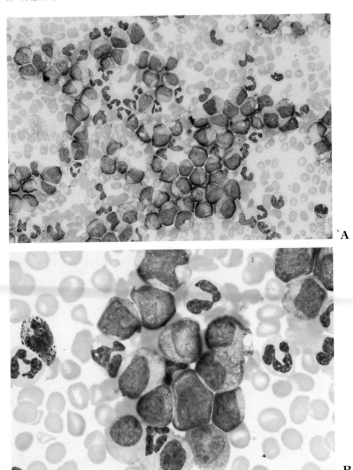

A

B

27. These are low (A) and high power (B) photographs of the blood film of a middle-aged Moroccan woman with moderate anaemia whose spleen was palpable 12 cm below the left costal margin.

a. Describe the abnormalities present.
b. What is the most likely diagnosis?
c. What cytogenetic abnormality would you expect to find?

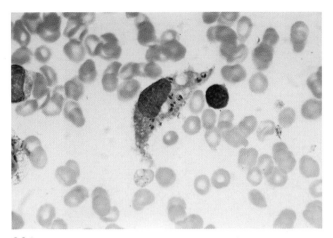

28. The slide shows bone marrow aspirate of a Maltese child who presented with fever and was found to have pancytopenia and slight splenomegaly.

a. What is the large cell in the centre?
b. What is the diagnosis?

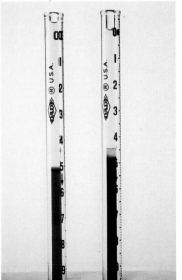

29. These haematocrit tubes are of a healthy control (left) and an elderly patient who presented with transient ischaemic attacks (right). The patient had a normal white cell count.

a. What abnormalities are shown?
b. What is the most likely diagnosis?
c. What is the likely cause of the transient ischaemic attacks?

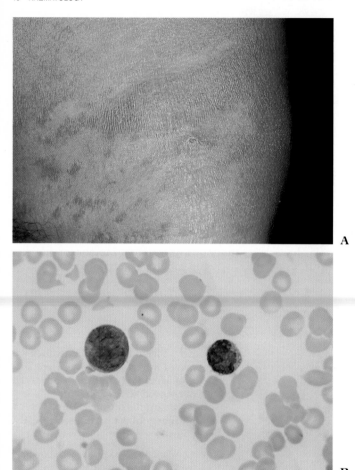

A

B

30. (A) shows the groin of an elderly man with a skin disorder, and (B) his blood film.

a. What is the most likely diagnosis?
b. What is the lineage of the two abnormal cells in the blood film?

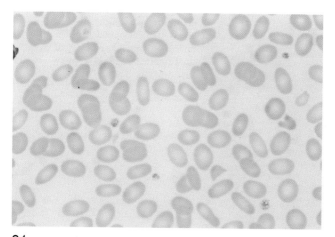

31. This is the blood film of a healthy young woman hospitalized for varicose vein surgery.

a. What is the diagnosis?
b. What is the clinical significance?

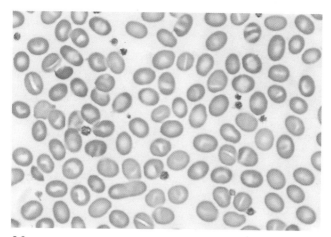

32. This is the blood film of a pregnant Malaysian woman with a haemoglobin concentration of 11.5 g/dl.

a. What is the diagnosis?
b. What is the clinical significance?

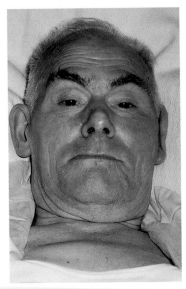

33. The photographs (A, B) show the face and foot of an elderly man. One toe had been amputated several years previously.

a. What is the most likely diagnosis?
b. List six tests that would be important in confirming the clinical diagnosis.

A

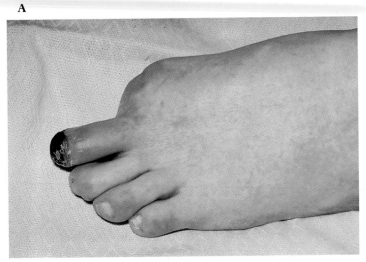

B

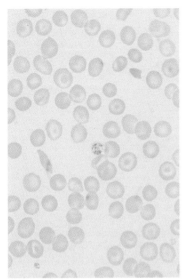

34. This is the blood film of a young Afro-Caribbean woman whose haemoglobin electrophoresis showed the following: haemoglobin S, 84.5%; haemoglobin A, 5%; haemoglobin A2, 3.5%; and haemoglobin F, 7%. The patient was pregnant and had never been transfused. Her haemoglobin concentration was 8.0 g/dl.

a. What abnormalities are shown in the blood film?
b. What is the diagnosis?
c. The patient's partner had sickle cell trait. What are the genetic implications?

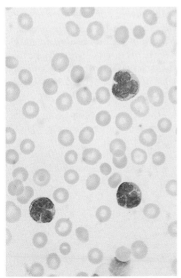

35. This is the blood film of a 36-year-old Afro-Caribbean male with generalized lymphadenopathy, cranial nerve palsies and hypercalcaemia. His blood count showed mild anaemia and thrombocytopenia.

a. Describe the abnormalities in the blood film.
b. What is the most likely diagnosis?
c. What aetiological agent is known for this condition?
d. What is the likely cause of the cranial nerve palsies?

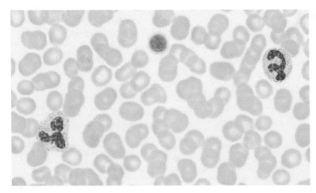

A

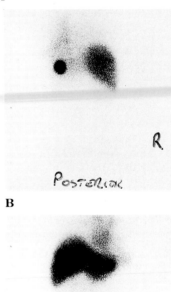

R

POSTERIOR

B

C

R   L

ANTERIOR

36. The slides show a peripheral blood film (A), two views of a radioisotopic scan after intravenous injection of heat-damaged technetium-labelled red cells (B, C), and a CT scan of the upper abdomen after oral contrast medium (D: opposite) from a young Asian woman with a past history of splenectomy for autoimmune thrombocytopenic purpura. Mucocutaneous bleeding had recommenced 2 months before these investigations. Bleeding was not ameliorated by high-dose corticosteroids.

a. Interpret the blood film in the light of the technetium scan.
b. Interpret the CT scan.
c. What further treatment might be offered to the patient?

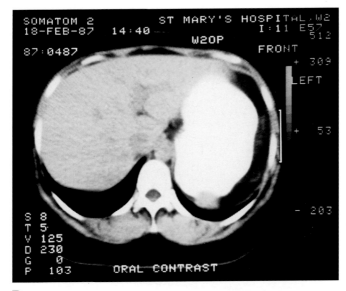

D

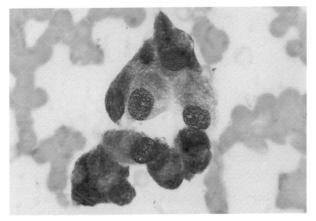

37. The slide shows a clump of cells in the bone marrow aspirate of a child being investigated following discovery of an abdominal mass.

a. What are the cells?
b. Are they any cause for concern?

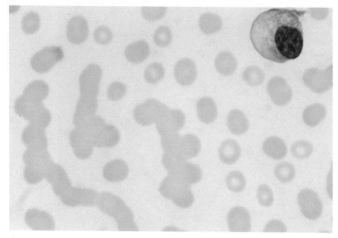

A

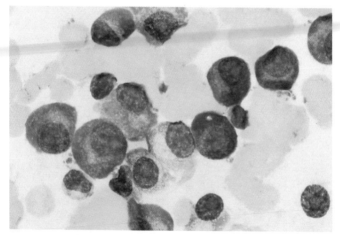

B

38. These are peripheral blood (A) and bone marrow (B) films from an elderly Caucasian male with bone pain, hypercalcaemia and mild renal impairment.

a. What is the most likely diagnosis?
b. What three further tests would be most useful in confirming the diagnosis?
c. What is the mechanism of the hypercalcaemia?

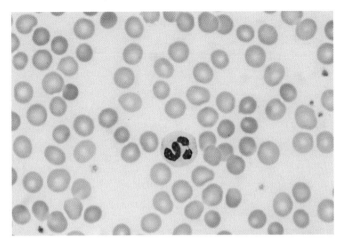

A

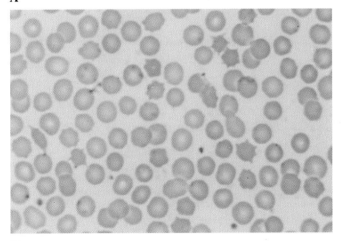

B

39. **These are blood films of a boy (A) and his father (B), both of whom have had episodic pallor and jaundice.**

a. What is the most likely diagnosis?
b. Why does the blood film of the father look different from that of the son?

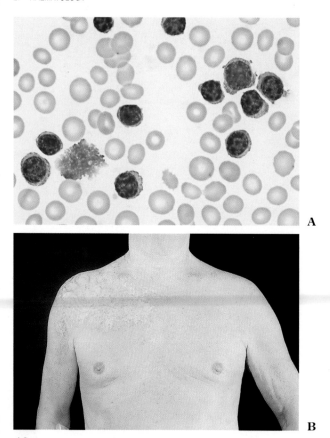

A

B

40. (A) is the blood film and (B) a clinical photograph of an elderly man with lymphadenopathy and hepatomegaly. He had been under treatment by a haematologist for 10 years. He had been treated with oral chemotherapy but not radiotherapy and his spleen had been removed.

a. Describe the abnormalities in the blood film.
b. What is the most likely diagnosis?
c. What single test would be most useful in confirming the diagnosis?
d. What is the likely cause of the abnormality shown in the clinical photograph?

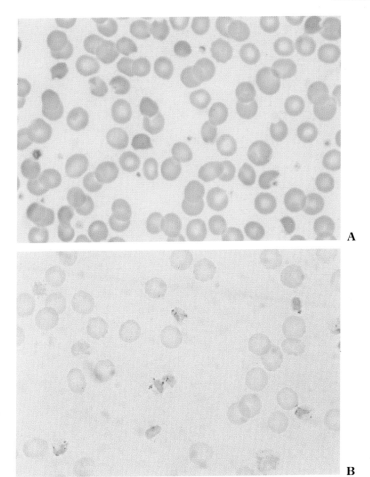

A

B

41. **This blood film (A) and this Heinz body preparation (B) are from a middle-aged Caucasian woman who is being treated for dermatitis herpetiformis and who is anaemic.**

a. What abnormality is shown in the blood film?
b. Explain the principle of the Heinz body test and state whether the test is positive or negative in this patient.
c. What is the nature of the anaemia and what is the likely cause?

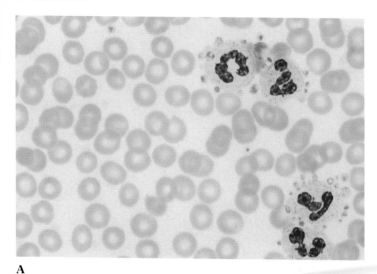

A

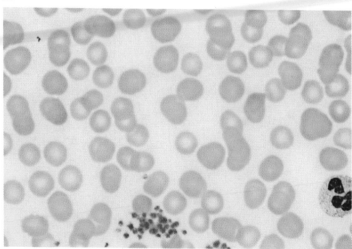

B

42. **These four blood films (A–D) are from patients with platelet counts on an automated blood cell counter of less than 20 × 10⁹/L.**

For each photograph, state what abnormality is shown and whether the platelet count is likely to be valid.

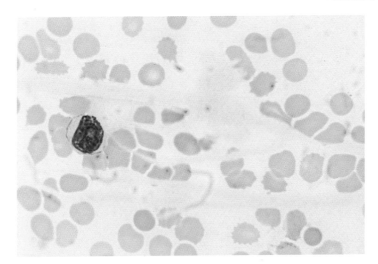

C

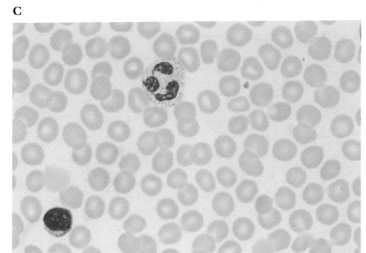

D

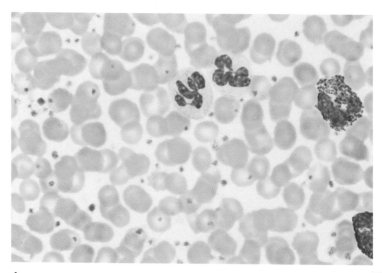

A

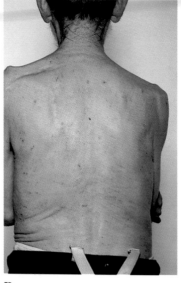

B

43. The blood film (A) and clinical photograph (B) are from an elderly Caucasian male with headaches, indigestion and a florid complexion.

a. What abnormality is shown by the blood film?
b. What is the most likely diagnosis?
c. What is the explanation of the abnormality shown in the photograph of the patient's back?

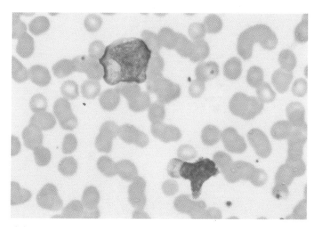

44. This is the blood film of a medical student with fever, pharyngitis, cervical lymphadenopathy and jaundice.

a. What abnormality is shown by the blood film?
b. What is the most likely diagnosis?
c. What test would be most useful to confirm the diagnosis?

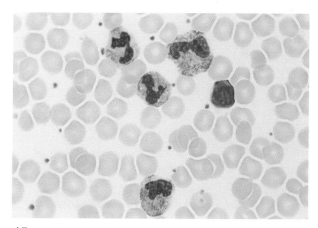

45. This is the blood film of a 63-year-old male with fever, cough and chest pain.

a. What abnormalities are shown?
b. How does the blood film contribute to the diagnosis?

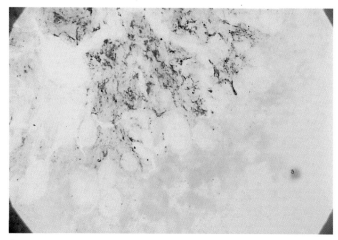

A

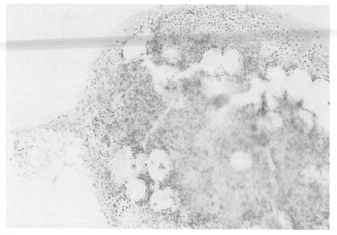

B

46. The slides (A, B) show bone marrow fragments from two patients stained with a Perls' stain for iron (Prussian blue reaction).

State whether each stain is positive or negative and explain the significance of the result.

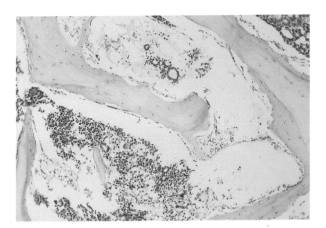

47. The slide shows a low power view of a trephine biopsy of bone marrow from a middle-aged man with urinary symptoms, hypercalcaemia and a leucoerythroblastic anaemia.

a   What does the histological section show?
b.   What is the most likely diagnosis?

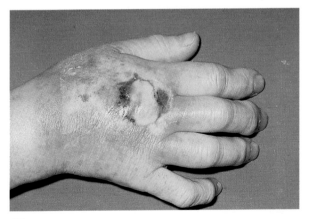

48. This is the hand of an elderly woman who has been having combination chemotherapy for a stage IV, high-grade non-Hodgkin's lymphoma.

a.   What abnormality is shown?
b.   What is the likely cause?

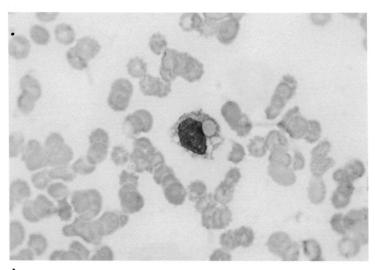

A

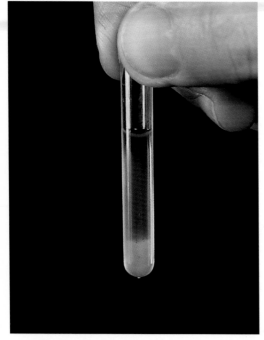

49. (A) is the blood film (prepared after cooling the blood) and (B) is a photograph of the chilled serum of a patient who suffered vascular symptoms in the hands and feet following exposure to cold.

a. What abnormality is shown?
b. What underlying diseases might provide an explanation?

B

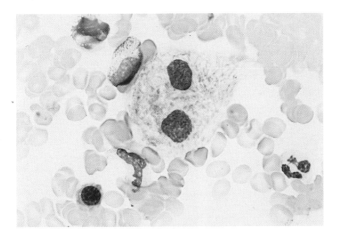

50. **This bone marrow aspirate is from a 42-year-old male with pancytopenia and moderate splenomegaly.**

What is the diagnosis?

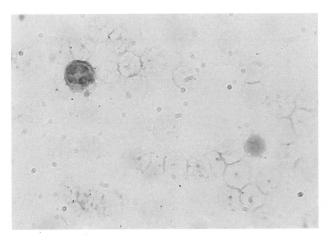

51. **The slide shows a Kleihauer test performed on a Rhesus-negative woman who had recently given birth.**

a. Explain the principle of the test.
b. State whether this test result indicates that a feto-maternal haemorrhage has occurred.

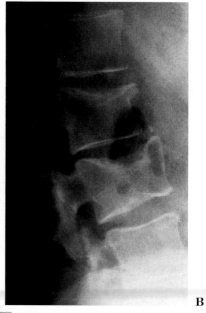

A

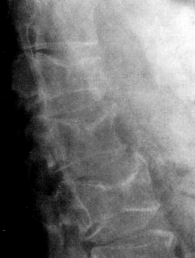

C

52. These are serial radiographs of the lumbar spine of a middle-aged man with back pain and anaemia taken at 1 year intervals (A–C). During this period the patient was receiving chemotherapy.

a. What abnormality is shown by the radiographs?
b. What is the most likely diagnosis?

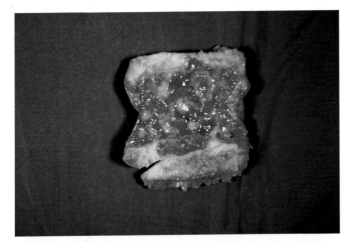

A

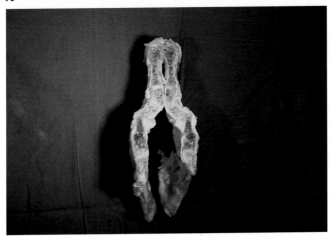

B

53. **(A) and (B) are photographs of a lumbar vertebra and of the sternum, respectively, at autopsy from the same patient as in question 52.**

a. What abnormality is shown by the vertebra?
b. What abnormality is shown by the sternum?

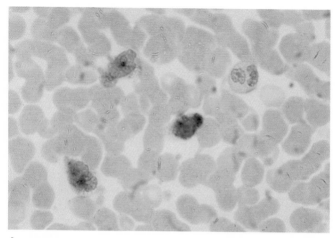

A

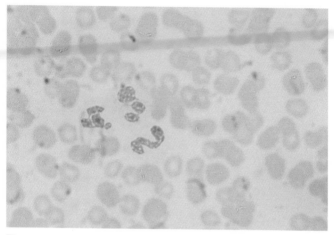

B

54. These are neutrophil alkaline phosphatase stains (also referred to as leucocyte alkaline phosphatase stains) from a healthy control subject (A) and a patient in whom a diagnosis of chronic granulocytic leukaemia was suspected (B).

Interpret the reaction in the patient and state how it contributes to the diagnosis.

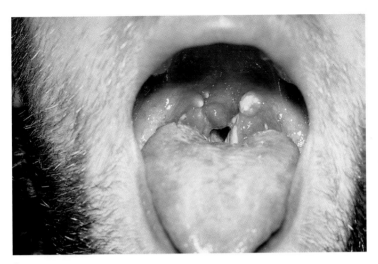

A

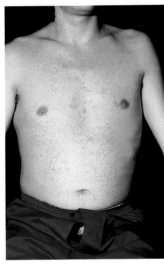

B

55. These are clinical photographs of the throat (A) and trunk (B) of a 35-year-old man presenting with an acute febrile illness. The blood film count was as follows: white cell count, 17 × 10⁹/L; haemoglobin concentration, 13.7 g/dl; platelet count, 110 × 10⁹/L; neutrophil count, 8.6 × 10⁹/L; and lymphocyte count, 7.0 × 10⁹/L. The blood film showed atypical lymphocytes.

a. What abnormality is shown by the throat?
b. What abnormality is shown by the trunk?
c. What is the most likely diagnosis?
d. What is the cause of this condition?

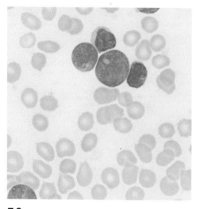 A

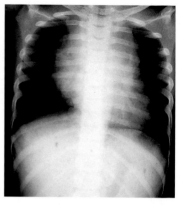 B

56. (A) and (B) are the blood film and chest X-ray of a 6-year-old boy with pallor and marked cervical lymphadenopathy.

a. What cells are shown in the blood?
b. What is the most likely diagnosis?
c. What abnormality is shown in the chest X-ray?
d. In view of the chest X-ray findings, what is the most likely lineage of the cells?

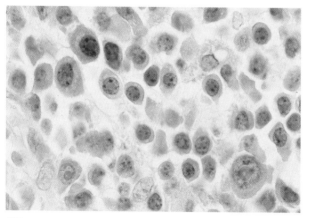 A

57. The three slides show histological sections stained with haematoxylin and eosin (H&E) (A) and by an immunoperoxidase technique with an antibody to kappa light chain (B, opposite) and lambda light chain (C, opposite).

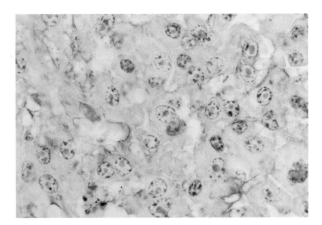

B

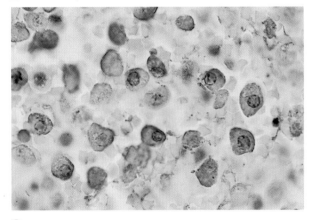

C

a. What does the H&E-stained section show?
b. Give an interpretation of the immunohistochemistry.
c. What is the diagnosis?

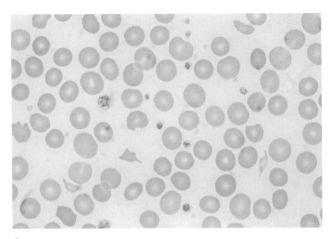

A

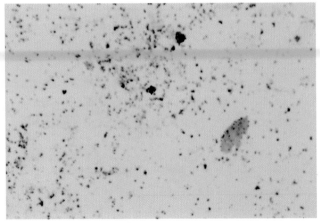

B

58. **The slides show the blood film (A) and urinary haemosiderin preparation (B) of an anaemic patient with a prosthetic mitral valve which has recently developed a perivalvular leak.**

a. What abnormality is shown by the blood film?
b. Is the test for urinary haemosiderin positive or negative?
c. What is the likely cause of the anaemia?

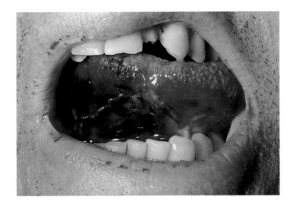

59. This is the mouth of a middle-aged man with a normal prothrombin time and thrombin time and a prolonged activated partial thromboplastin time.

What is the most likely diagnosis?

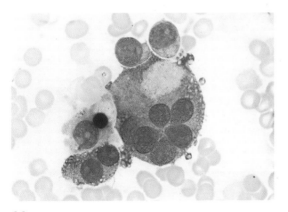

60. This bone marrow film is from an elderly woman with a recent onset of bruising and fatigue. Slight splenomegaly was detected and the blood count showed pancytopenia. Her blood film showed anisocytosis, poikilocytosis and the presence of hypogranular neutrophils.

a. What morphological abnormalities are shown?
b. What is the most likely diagnosis?

Coagulation test results

Prothrombin time	38 s (normal range, 14.5–19.5)
Activated partial thromboplastin time	80 s (normal range, 28–32)
Thrombin time	40 s (control, 13)
Fibrinogen	0.8 g/L (normal range, 1.4–3.5)
FDPs	40 mg/L (normal range, <10)

A

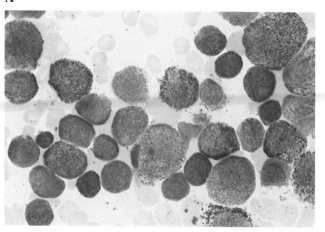

B

61. These coagulation test results (A) and the bone marrow aspirate (B) are from a 23-year-old man who presented with a recent onset of bruising.

a. What does the bone marrow film show?
b. How do you interpret the coagulation tests?
c. What is your final diagnosis?
d. What cytogenetic abnormality would you expect?

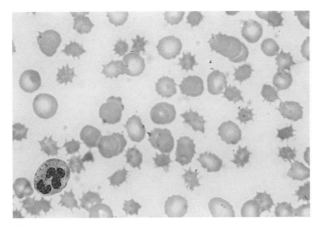

62. This blood film is from a patient with liver failure.

a. What abnormality is shown?
b. Is this of any clinical significance?

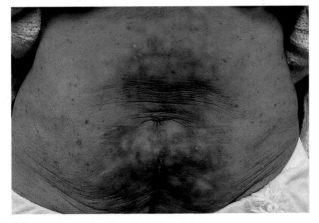

63. This is the abdomen of a West Indian woman with a previous history of Hodgkin's disease who is now suffering from weight loss and night sweats. An abdominal CT scan was normal 2 months previously. There is a past history of hysterectomy.

a. What abnormalities are present?
b. What is the most likely explanation?

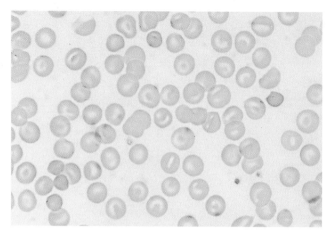

A

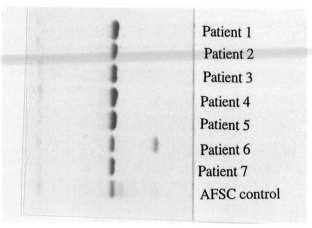

Patient 1
Patient 2
Patient 3
Patient 4
Patient 5
Patient 6
Patient 7
AFSC control

B

64. These slides show the blood film (A) and haemoglobin electrophoresis on cellulose acetate at alkaline pH (B) of a healthy Afro-Caribbean woman (Patient 6) with a haemoglobin concentration of 12.7 g/dl and an MCV of 78 fl.

a. What abnormalities are shown in the blood film?
b. What is the likely diagnosis?

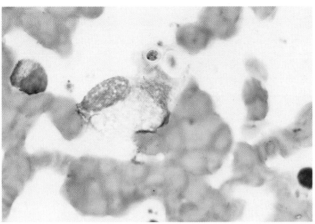

A

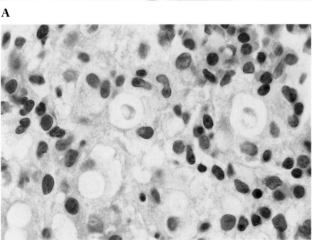

B

65. These slides show the bone marrow aspirate and trephine biopsy from a young man with advanced HIV infection.

What abnormality is shown?

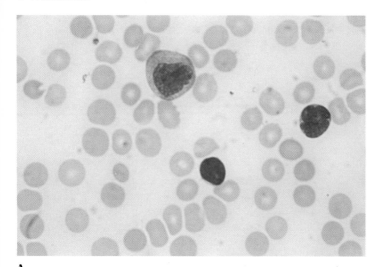

A

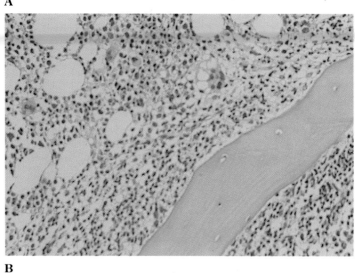

B

66. The blood film (A), trephine biopsy (B) and low and high power views of a lymph node (C, D: opposite) are from a 63-year-old man with generalized lymphadenopathy and mild hepatosplenomegaly.

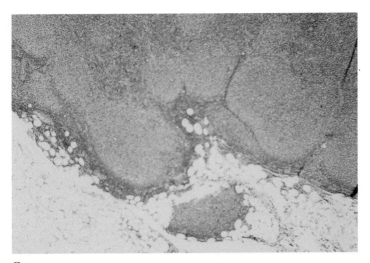

C

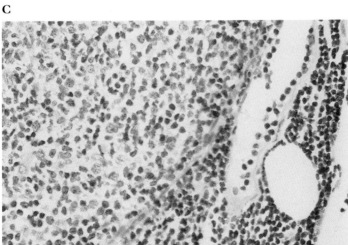

D

a. Describe the significant abnormalities.

b. What is the diagnosis?

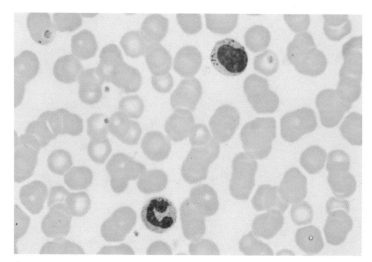

A

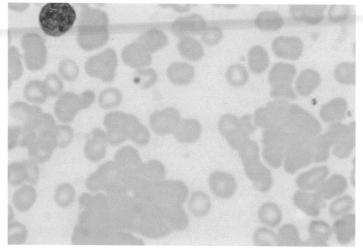

B

67. These blood films are from two patients.

a. What abnormality is shown in (A) and what is its significance?
b. What abnormality is shown in (B) and what is its significance?

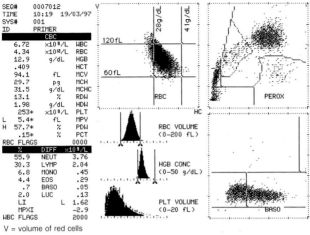

SEQ#	0007012	
TIME	10:19	19/03/97
SYS#	001	
ID	PRIMER	

CBC

6.72	×10⁹/L	WBC
4.34	×10¹²/L	RBC
12.9	g/dL	HGB
.409		HCT
94.1	fL	MCV
29.7	pg	MCH
31.5	g/dL	MCHC
13.1	%	RDW
1.98	g/dL	HDW
253*	×10⁹/L	PLT
L 5.4*	fL	MPV
H 57.7*	%	PDW
.15*	%	PCT
RBC FLAGS		0000

%	DIFF	×10⁹/L
55.9	NEUT	3.76
30.3	LYMP	2.04
6.8	MONO	.45
4.4	EOS	.29
.7	BASO	.05
2.0	LUC	.13
	LI	L 1.62
	MPXI	-2.9
WBC FLAGS		2000

V = volume of red cells
HC = haemoglobin corcentration

A

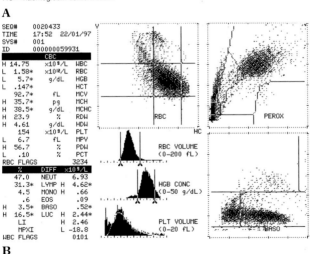

SEQ#	0020433	
TIME	17:52	22/01/97
SYS#	001	
ID	000000059931	

CBC

H 14.75	×10⁹/L	WBC
L 1.58*	×10¹²/L	RBC
L 5.7*	g/dL	HGB
L .147*		HCT
92.7*	fL	MCV
H 35.7*	pg	MCH
H 38.5*	g/dL	MCHC
H 23.9	%	RDW
H 4.61	g/dL	HDW
154	×10⁹/L	PLT
L 6.7	fL	MPV
H 56.7	%	PDW
L .10	%	PCT
RBC FLAGS		3234

%	DIFF	×10⁹/L
47.0	NEUT	6.93
31.3*	LYMP H	4.62*
4.5	MONO H	.66
.6	EOS	.09
H 3.5*	BASO	.52*
H 16.5*	LUC H	2.44*
	LI	H 2.46
	MPXI	L -18.8
WBC FLAGS		0101

B

68. These automated printouts from a Bayer–Technicon H.2 automated counter were obtained from a healthy subject (**A**) and from a patient whose blood film is shown in question 67(**B**) and who reported red urine after being exposed to the cold (**B**).

a. What abnormalities are shown in the printout of the patient's blood?
b. What is the clinical significance?

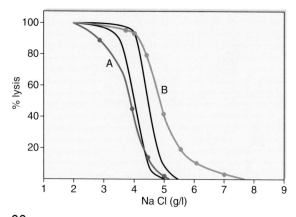

69. This is an osmotic fragility test showing results in two patients (A, B) with congenital haemolytic anaemia. The normal range is also indicated.

Interpret both results.

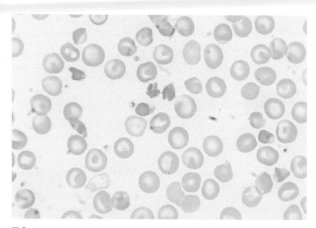

70. This is the blood film of a west African patient with a positive sickle solubility test.

a. What abnormalities are shown?
b. What is the likely diagnosis?
c. What significance, if any, would this diagnosis have?

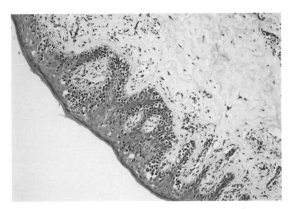

A

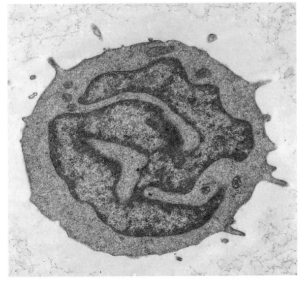

B

71. (A) is a skin biopsy and (B) is an electron micrography of a peripheral blood lymphocyte from a patient whose skin showed erythematous patches and thickened plaques and nodules.

a. What abnormalities are shown?
b. What is the diagnosis?

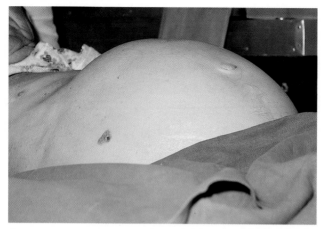

A

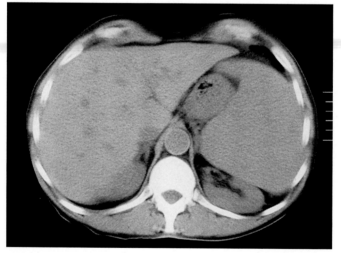

B

72. **(A) shows the abdomen of one patient and (B) is a CT scan of another patient, both of whom have pancytopenia and a leucoerythroblastic blood film. Both patients have the same disease.**

a. Describe the abnormalities present.
b. What is the most likely diagnosis?

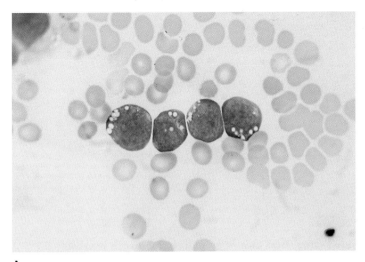

A

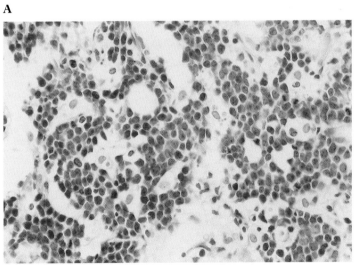

B

73. **These slides show a bone marrow film (A) and a lymph node biopsy (B).**

What is the diagnosis?

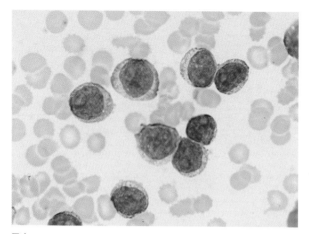

74. This is the blood film of an elderly man with marked splenomegaly.

What is the most likely diagnosis?

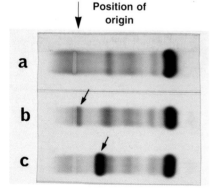

Position of origin

a

b

c

75. The slide shows electrophoresis or serum proteins in blood of a normal volunteer (a) and two patients (b, c).

a. What abnormality is shown in patient b?
b. What abnormality is shown in patient c?
c. What disease is most likely to cause these abnormalities?

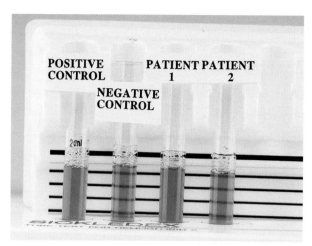

A

B

76. (A) is a sickle solubility test showing a positive control, a negative control, and patients 1 and 2. (B) is a haemoglobin electrophoresis on cellulose acetate at alkaline pH.

a. What is the diagnosis in patient 1?
b. What is the most likely diagnosis in patient 2?

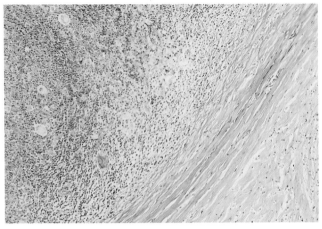

A

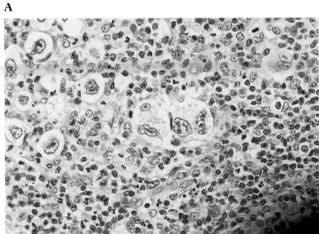

B

77. These slides show a lymph node biopsy at low and high power
(A, B), stained, respectively, with a Giemsa stain and with
haematoxylin and eosin, and a lymph node imprint stained with a
May–Grünwald–Giemsa stain (C: opposite).

a. What is the diagnosis?
b. What is the large cell in the lymph node imprint?

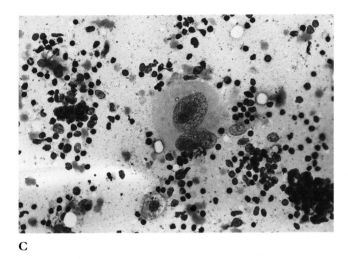

C

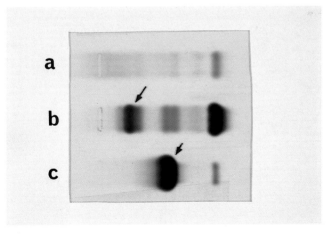

78. **This slide shows a urinary electrophoresis in three patients with multiple myeloma.**

a. Give an interpretation of a.
b. Give an interpretation of b.
c. Give an interpretation of c.

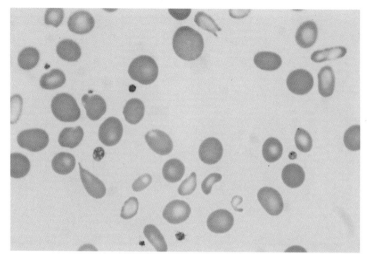

A

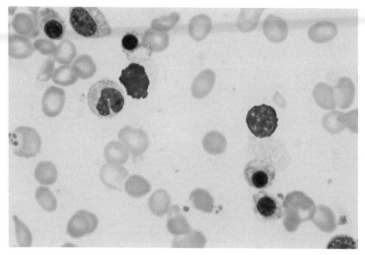

B

79. (A) is a peripheral blood film, (B) is a bone marrow aspirate stained with May–Grünwald–Giemsa stain, and (C) and (D) are low and high power views, respectively, of an iron stain of the bone marrow of an elderly anaemic man.

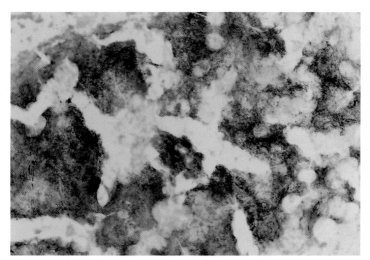

C

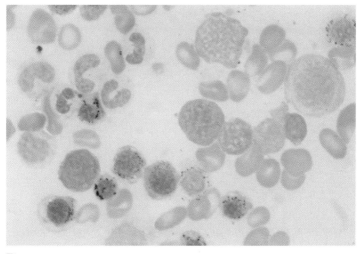

D

a. What abnormalities are shown in the blood film?
b. What abnormality is shown in the bone marrow aspirate?
c. What abnormalities are shown in the iron stains?
d. What is the final diagnosis?

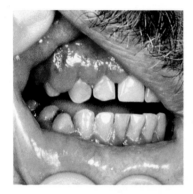

A

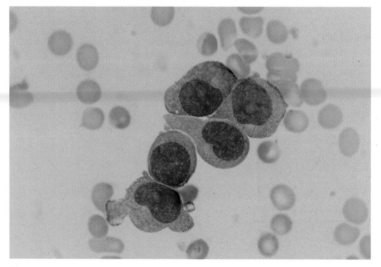

B

80. These photographs are of the mouth (A) and bone marrow aspirate (B) of two patients with the same diagnosis.

a. What abnormalities are shown in the mouth and on the bone marrow aspirate?
b. What is the diagnosis?

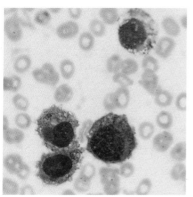
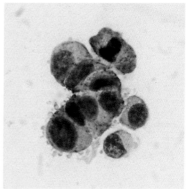

A   **B**

81. This bone marrow aspirate is from a 42-year-old woman with a leucoerythroblastic anaemia, stained by May–Grünwald–Giemsa stain (A) and by an immunocytochemical technique with a monoclonal antibody to cytokeratin (B).

a. What do the photographs show?
b. What is the diagnosis?

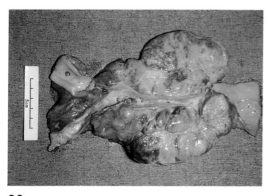

82. This is an autopsy specimen showing the aorta and para-aortic lymph nodes.

a. What abnormality is shown?
b. What are the most likely diagnoses?

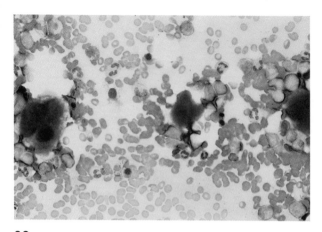

83. This is a low power view of a bone marrow aspirate from a patient with recent onset of severe thrombocytopenia in whom the diagnosis of autoimmune thrombocytopenic purpura is suspected.

a. Describe the findings.
b. Does this bone marrow aspirate support the diagnosis?

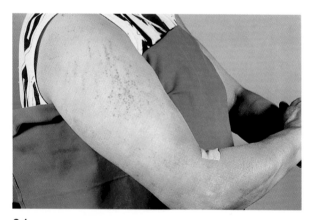

84. This is a patient's arm.

a. What abnormality is shown?
b. Give two possible explanations.

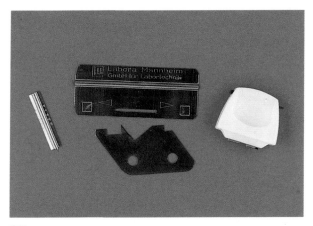

85. The devices shown are used for a haematology test.

What test are they used for?

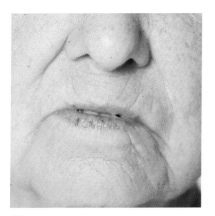

86. This is the mouth of a patient who has had recurrent nose bleeds since the age of 20, and more recently recurrent gastrointestinal haemorrhage.

What is the diagnosis?

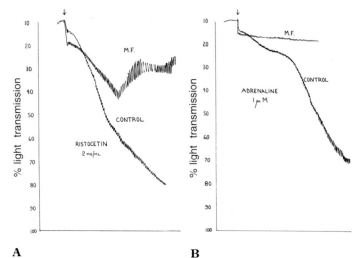

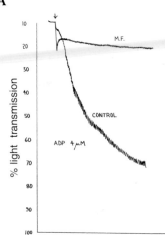

87. (A)–(C) show platelet aggregation studies in a young girl who has suffered recurrent epistaxes of such severity that blood transfusion has sometimes been necessary. The platelet count and the blood film were normal.

a. What abnormality is shown?
b. What is the most likely diagnosis?

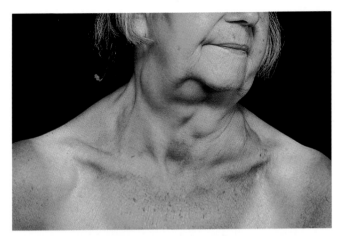

A

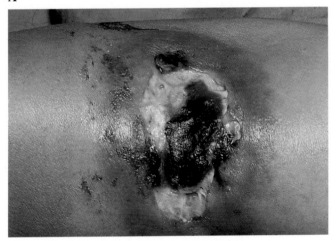

B

88. These photographs show two patients with the same diagnosis. Both had anaemia and lymphocytosis. The lesion shown in (B) is the result of a smallpox vaccination.

a. Describe the abnormality shown in (A).
b. Describe the abnormality shown in (B).
c. What single disease would explain the abnormalities?

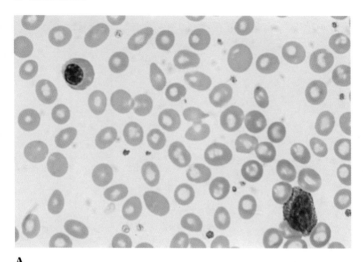

A

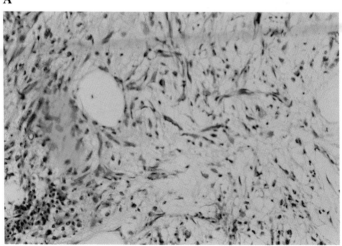

B

89. (A) is a peripheral blood film and (B) and (C) are low power views of a bone marrow trephine biopsy from a middle-aged male with pancytopenia and splenomegaly. The trephine biopsy is stained with haematoxylin and eosin (B) and for reticulin (C). A reticulin stain of a normal trephine biopsy is shown for comparison (D).

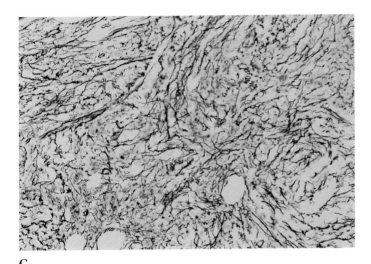

C

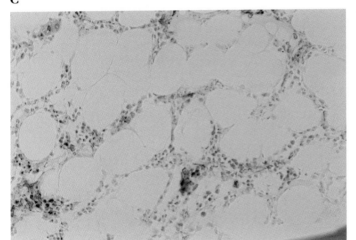

D

a. Describe the abnormalities.
b. What is the likely diagnosis?

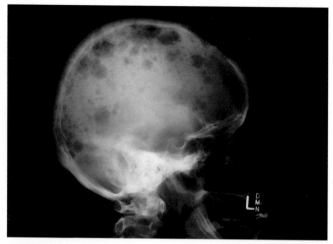

A

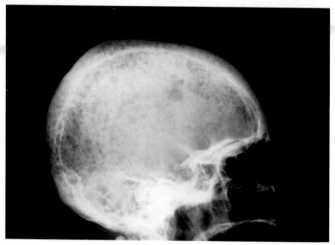

B

90. **(A) and (B) are skull X-rays from two patients with the same disease. The patient in (B) also suffers from a second disease.**

a. What disease does the patient shown in (A) suffer from?
b. What two diseases does the patient shown in (B) suffer from?

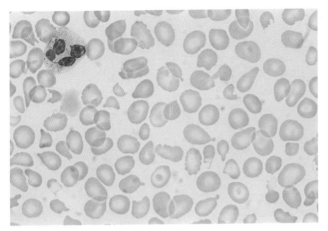

A

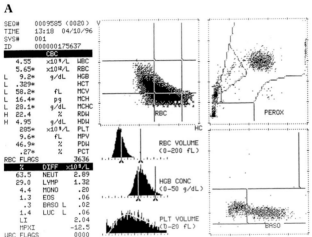

B

91. (A) is a peripheral blood film and (B) an automated full blood count and red cell cytogram (Bayer–Technicon H.2 automated counter) from a Cypriot patient with splenomegaly.

a. What abnormalities are shown in the blood film and count?
b. Compare the red cell cytogram with the normal cytogram in question 68 and describe the abnormalities that are present.
c. What is the most likely diagnosis?

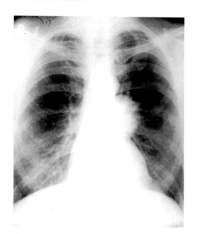
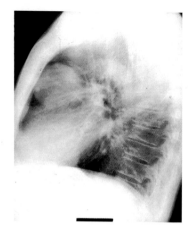

92. These are PA and lateral chest X-rays in a patient with pure red cell aplasia.

a. What abnormality is shown?
b. What is the nature of the red cell aplasia?

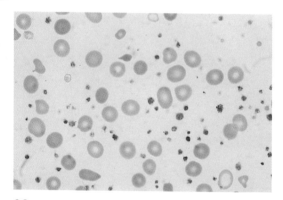

93. This is the blood film of a patient with a 10 year history of essential thrombocythaemia which had been treated on several occasions with ^{32}P. She now has a haemoglobin concentration of 7.3 g/dl.

a. Has the thrombocythaemia been well controlled?
b. What abnormalities are shown in the blood film?
c. What is the possible mechanism of the haematological abnormalities?

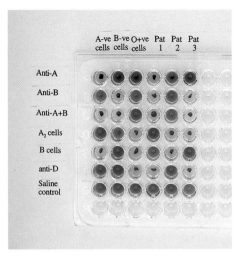

94. This is a blood grouping reaction showing the reactions of anti-A, anti-B, anti-A+B and anti-D with control cells and cells from three patients, together with reactions of the patients' serum with A2 cells and B cells.

a. what is the blood group of patient 1?
b. What is the blood group of patient 2?
c. What is the blood group of patient 3?

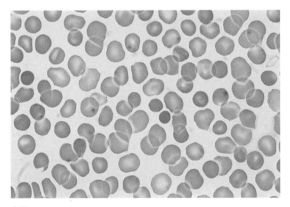

95. This is the blood film of a jaundiced neonate. The baby is of blood group A and the mother is blood group O. Both are Rhesus D positive.

a. What abnormality is shown in the blood film?
b. What is the most likely diagnosis?

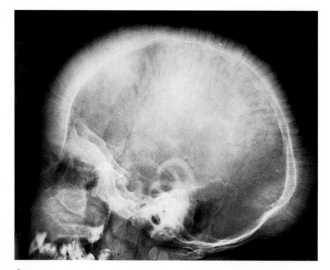

A

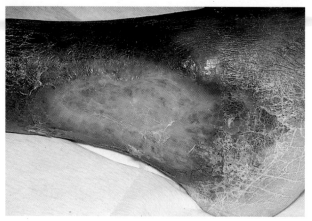

B

96. (A) is a skull X-ray and (B) a clinical photograph of two patients with the same disease.

a. Describe the abnormalities.
b. What disease is most likely to cause these abnormalities?

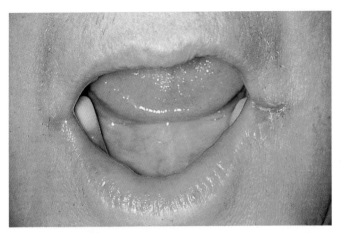

A

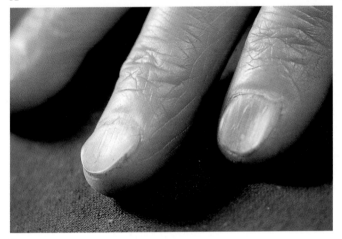

B

97. **These clinical photographs are of two patients with the same diagnosis.**

a. What abnormality is shown in (A)?
b. What abnormality is shown in (B)?
c. What is the underlying condition that causes both these abnormalities?

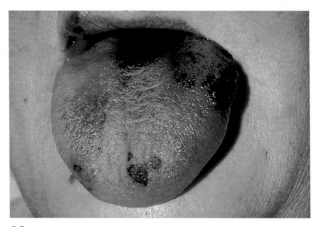

98. **This is the mouth of a 30-year-old woman with a recent sudden onset of nose bleeds and bruising.**

a. What is the most likely haematological diagnosis?

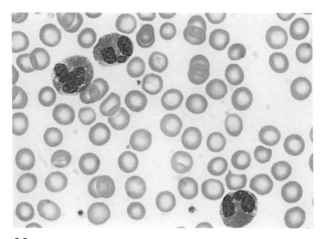

99. **This is a blood film.**

a. Identify the three leucocytes.
b. Give three causes of an increase in this cell type.

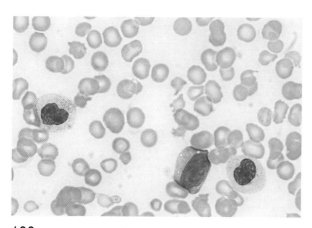

100. This is the blood film of an elderly woman with a past history of polycythaemia rubra vera who had been treated by venesection and with ^{32}P.

a. What abnormalities are shown?
b. What is the likely explanation?

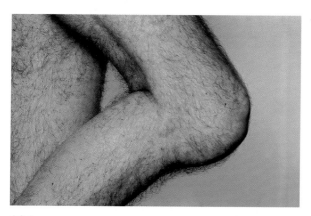

101. This is the knee of an adult male photographed 20 years ago. His older brother was similarly affected.

a. What is the most likely haematological diagnosis?
b. Why are such clinical manifestations much less likely to be seen nowadays?

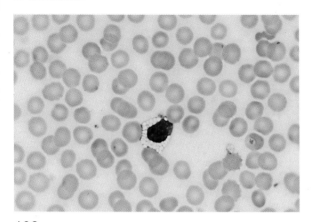

102. This is a peripheral blood cell from a 2-year-old child with short stature, psychomotor retardation, mild hepatosplenomegaly and gum hyperplasia, with widely spaced ill-formed teeth.

a. Identify the cell and the abnormality.
b. Give three causes of this morphological abnormality.

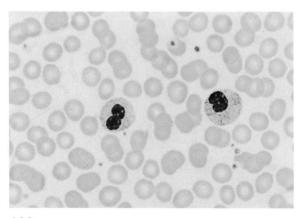

103. This blood film is from a healthy 40-year-old man attending surgical outpatients for assessment of an inguinal hernia. His blood count was normal.

a. What abnormality is shown?
b. What is the clinical significance?

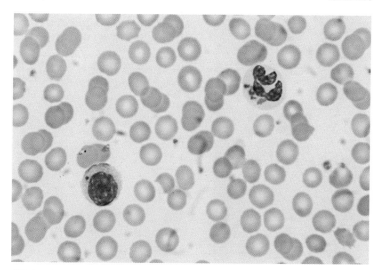

104. This is a peripheral blood film of an 8-year-old child with partial oculocutaneous albinism, recurrent infections, hepatosplenomegaly, lymphadenopathy and thrombocytopenia.

a. What is the morphological abnormality?
b. What is the diagnosis?

Result of acidified serum test

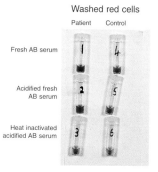

Washed red cells

Patient   Control

Fresh AB serum

Acidified fresh AB serum

Heat inactivated acidified AB serum

105. This is an acid lysis test in a patient with pancytopenia and a history of passing red urine.

a. Explain the test and state whether it is positive or negative.
b. What is the likely diagnosis?

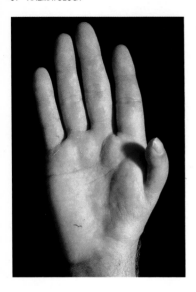

106. **This is the hand of a child with gradual onset of pancytopenia.**

a. What abnormality is shown?
b. What is the most likely diagnosis?

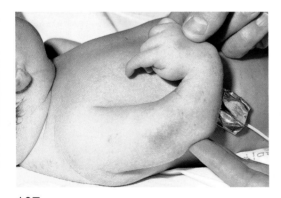

107. **This is the arm of a young child with thrombocytopenia.**

a. What abnormality is shown?
b. What is the diagnosis?

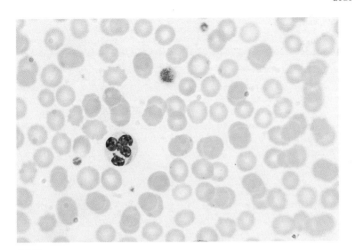

108. This is the blood film of a young man with a history of life-long mild bruising.

a. What three abnormalities are shown?
b. What is the most likely diagnosis?

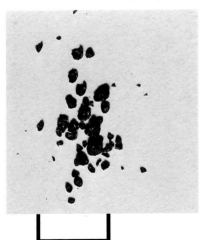

1cm

109. These are gallstones which were removed surgically.

a. What is the nature of the gallstones?
b. What underlying disease is likely?

Answers

1. a. The blood film shows basophilic stippling. This is consequent on abnormal staining of ribosomal RNA. It is a non-specific feature which is common in dyserythropoietic conditions. Basophilic stippling is particularly prominent in patients with an inherited deficiency of a red cell enzyme, pyrimidine 5′ nucleotidase. It is also common in lead poisoning in which the function of this enzyme is inhibited by lead.
   b. The gums show a lead line, consequent on deposition of lead.
   c. The findings are those of lead poisoning. This diagnosis was confirmed by the demonstration of an increased serum lead concentration—82 µg/100 ml (normal range, <40). Lead poisoning can cause a hypochromic microcytic anaemia or, as in this patient, a haemolytic anaemia. The increased reticulocyte count is consequent on the increased rate of red cell breakdown. Patients of Indian ethnic origin sometimes suffer from lead poisoning because of lead in cosmetics, but in this patient the cause of the lead poisoning could not be identified.

2. a. The most significant abnormality is the presence of sickle cells.
   b. The most likely diagnosis is sickle cell anaemia, i.e. homozygosity for haemoglobin S. It should be noted that the term sickle cell disease is used more broadly and includes conditions such as compound heterozygosity for haemoglobin S and haemoglobin C, and compound heterozygosity for haemoglobin S and β-thalassaemia. In this patient, homozygosity for haemoglobin S is more likely than sickle cell/haemoglobin C disease because the sickle cells are quite numerous and, in addition, it is the commoner condition. Sickle cell/β-thalassaemia compound heterozygosity is associated with microcytosis as a consequence of a reduced rate of synthesis of β-globin chains, and in this patient is excluded by the normal MCV.
   c. The test that should be performed is haemoglobin electrophoresis. If the patient is homozygous for haemoglobin S, electrophoresis would show mainly haemoglobin S with a small amount of haemoglobin A_2 and possibly an increased proportion of haemoglobin F. There would be no haemoglobin A. A sickle solubility test is also usually

performed in any patient with a variant haemoglobin with the mobility of haemoglobin S, in order to distinguish haemoglobin S from non-sickling variant haemoglobins such as haemoglobin D and haemoglobin G, which have the same mobility as haemoglobin S at alkaline pH. The sickle solubility test would be positive in this patient but the test could be considered to be redundant since sickle cells are clearly present in the blood film.

d. One of the three platelets present is increased in size. This is likely to be a feature of the hyposplenism which is usually present in adults with sickle cell anaemia, consequent on previous splenic infarction.

3.
a. There are four reticulocytes.

b. The reticulocyte count is increased. There are about 80 red cells in the photograph. If the photograph is representative then the reticulocyte count is about 5%, i.e. about twice the normal level. An elevated reticulocyte count could be consequent on haemolysis or recent haemorrhage, or could be a response to iron, vitamin B_{12} or folic acid administered to a patient deficient in one of these haematinics. A reticulocyte stain is referred to as a vital or supravital stain because the red cells are not fixed before exposure to the dye. The stain interacts with the RNA of any residual ribosomes, causing them to precipitate and take up the stain.

4.
a. The blood film shows two gametocytes of *Plasmodium falciparum*. Note that the cells containing the parasites contain no visible haemoglobin.

b. The diagnosis is malaria due to *Plasmodium falciparum*, otherwise known as malignant tertian malaria.

5.
a. The skin changes are those of vitiligo. The patient has been treated with UV light and the abnormality is therefore quite striking.

b. Patients with vitiligo show an increased incidence of pernicious anaemia.

6.
a. The smaller cell is a blast cell containing an Auer rod. The other intact cell is an abnormal myeloid cell. The slide also shows a crushed cell, known as a smear cell.

b. The likely diagnosis is acute myeloid leukaemia. Auer rods are crystalline structures derived from the primary granules of myeloid cells. They are specific for acute myeloid leukaemia and the closely related myelodysplastic syndromes. Considering the age of the patient, the clinical features, the blood count and the presence of a blast cell containing an Auer rod, a diagnosis of acute myeloid leukaemia is more likely than a diagnosis of one of the myelodysplastic syndromes. The presence of smear cells indicates that cells have increased mechanical fragility. Such cells are characteristic of chronic lymphocytic leukaemia, but they may be seen in many other conditions.

7.

a. The blood count shows anaemia, microcytosis and a reduced mean cellular haemoglobin concentration.

b. The two most significant abnormalities in the film are hypochromia and microcytosis. There is also anisocytosis and poikilocytosis, and it is apparent that the patient is anaemic. However, these latter abnormalities are less specific with regard to diagnosis. Anaemia can be detected in a blood film because the reduced haemoglobin concentration leads to reduced viscosity of the blood, which in turn means that the film of blood is spread more thinly on the glass slide and the red cells are further apart. Hypochromia is present because the area of central pallor is about two-thirds of the diameter of the red cell rather than the normal one-third. Microcytosis is detected by noting that the diameter of the red cells, in relation to the neutrophil, is reduced. Anaemia and microcytosis are thus shown by both the blood count and the film. The hypochromia shown by the blood film is reflected in the reduced MCHC shown by the blood count.

c. The most likely diagnosis is iron deficiency anaemia.

d. The diagnosis could be confirmed by demonstrating either a reduced serum ferritin concentration or the combination of a reduced serum iron concentration and an increase in either the iron binding capacity or the serum transferrin concentration. It is important to remember that a reduced serum iron concentration is, by itself, of little use in diagnosis since this will also be seen in patients with the anaemia of chronic disease who are likely to have either normal or increased bone marrow iron stores. Measuring transferrin or iron binding capacity is more useful because these measurements are usually increased in iron deficiency and decreased in the anaemia of chronic disease.

e. It is important to investigate this patient for gastrointestinal bleeding, e.g. from carcinoma of the colon. In view of his symptoms, bleeding is more likely to be from the lower than the upper gastrointestinal tract, so either a colonoscopy or a barium enema would be an appropriate initial investigation. It should be noted that a man of this age with a normal diet and an iron deficiency anaemia should be investigated for blood loss even if there are no gastrointestinal symptoms.

8.
a. The film shows anaemia, anisocytosis, poikilocytosis and the presence of macrocytes.
b. The most significant abnormalities are the presence of macrocytes and, in particular, the presence of oval macrocytes. The latter suggest that the patient may have a megaloblastic anaemia.
c. The most likely diagnosis, considering both the patient's age and the presence of neurological symptoms, is pernicious anaemia. Weight loss and loss of appetite are fairly common in patients with severe megaloblastic anaemia and do not necessarily indicate that anaemia is caused by dietary folic acid deficiency.

9.
a. The blood film shows anaemia, severe thrombocytopenia (only one platelet visible), red cell fragments and one polychromatic macrocyte.
b. Anaemia with red cell fragments is indicative of a microangiopathic haemolytic anaemia. The polychromatic macrocyte suggests that a reticulocyte response is occurring.
c. In view of the oliguria, elevated creatinine and microangiopathic haemolytic anaemia, the likely diagnosis is haemolytic-uraemic syndrome consequent on infection by verocytotoxin-secreting *E. coli*. This is now the commonest cause of acute renal failure in children in the UK. The presence of severe thrombocytopenia raises the possibility of thrombotic thrombocytopenia purpura, which can also follow *E. coli* infection. This name is given to a syndrome of fever, microangiopathic haemolytic anaemia, thrombocytopenia and neurological symptoms caused by a microangiopathy with platelet consumption and small vessel obstruction.

10.
a. Three of the cells are monocytes, and the other is a neutrophil. The neutrophil is hypogranular.
b. The patient had chronic myelomonocytic leukaemia. This condition is usually classified as one of the myelodysplastic syndromes because the cells often show some morphological abnormalities (dysplastic features) and haemopoiesis is to some extent ineffective (reduced production of mature cells of some lineages despite a cellular bone marrow).

11.
a. The haematocrit is 0.50 in the tube on the left and 0.56 in the tube on the right.
b. The white band above the red cell column is referred to as the 'buffy coat' and is composed mainly of white cells with some contribution from platelets. The size of the buffy coat in these two blood specimens shows that white cells were present in normal numbers.

12.
a. Erythropoiesis is megaloblastic and giant metamyelocytes are present. Megaloblastic erythropoiesis is characterized by large cells which have nuclei with a very open chromatin pattern; there is nucleocytoplasmic asynchrony with cytoplasm showing features of maturation (haemoglobinization and loss of basophilia) while the nucleus remains immature (delicate chromatin pattern with little condensation).

b. The diagnosis is megaloblastic anaemia, most likely due to deficiency of vitamin B_{12} or folic acid.

c. The most relevant initial tests would be assays of serum vitamin B_{12} and red cell folate concentrations. Serum folate assay would be less relevant, since serum folate reflects recent dietary intake whereas red cell folate reflects folic acid supply during the period when the red cells were being produced.

13.
a. The central film shows a marked increase in uptake of the basic component of the stain, conveying a deep blue colour to the film.

b. Such abnormal staining characteristics are usually indicative of a marked increase in plasma proteins, most often as a consequence of multiple myeloma.

14.
The blood film shows striking stomatocytosis. In addition, two cells show basophilic stippling. This patient has a rare inherited haemolytic anaemia known as hereditary stomatocytosis. Commoner causes of stomatocytosis are alcoholic liver disease and macrocytosis associated with hydroxyurea therapy.

15.
a. The film shows severe thrombocytopenia (only a single platelet) and a marked increase in platelet size.

b. The syndrome comprising thrombocytopenia, giant platelets, sensorineural deafness and renal insufficiency is inherited and is referred to as Epstein's syndrome. It has an autosomal inheritance and is a variant of Alport's syndrome which is characterized by nephritis and deafness.

16.
a. The chest X-ray shows superior mediastinal widening which is likely to be indicative of mediastinal lymphadenopathy.

b. The most likely diagnosis is Hodgkin's disease.

17.
a. The blood film shows large numbers of nucleated red cells, target cells, Pappenheimer bodies, one spherocyte and one cell containing a small Howell–Jolly body. In addition, there are a considerable number of normal red cells which represent transfused cells. The transfused cells are normochromic, while the patient's cells are hypochromic. The film can therefore be referred to as dimorphic.

b. The diagnosis was beta-thalassaemia major. Features of hyposplenism are present. The presence of fairly numerous Pappenheimer bodies indicates the combined effect of hyposplenism and iron overload. A specific feature apparent in a red cell near the neutrophil is a condensed mass beneath the red cell membrane. This represents excess alpha chains which have precipitated because of the lack of beta chains able to combine with them.

18.
a. The blood film shows Howell–Jolly bodies and acanthocytes, indicating hyposplenism. There is only one platelet visible, indicating quite severe thrombocytopenia.
b. It is likely that the patient has been treated by splenectomy. This has either been ineffective or, if initially effective, it has been followed by relapse.

19.
a. The patient shows depilation, with the distribution suggesting that he has received mantle irradiation.
b. The patient suffered from Hodgkin's disease. This form of irradiation is often used for Hodgkin's disease, as the radiotherapy field includes the cervical, axillary and mediastinal lymph nodes (see diagram).

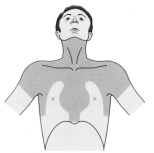

20.
The diagnosis is hairy cell leukaemia. Hairy cells are medium-sized lymphoid cells with plentiful, weakly basophilic ragged cytoplasm. Hairy cell leukaemia is characterized by splenomegaly and cytopenia, with monocytopenia being particularly prominent. The number of hairy cells in the blood is often quite low.

The cytochemical reaction shown is typical of hairy cell leukaemia. Hairy cells show tartrate-resistant acid phosphatase activity, whereas in most other cells acid phosphatase activity is inhibited by tartrate.

This is an important diagnosis to make as there are now drugs available (nucleoside analogues) which are very effective in the treatment of hairy cell leukaemia.

21.
a. Two trypanosomes are present (in this case *T. gambesiense*).
b. The disease caused is trypanosomiasis, or sleeping sickness.

22.
a. The haematocrit or packed cell volume is reduced, as red cells occupy only about a third of the total height of the column of blood. This indicates that the patient is anaemic.

If the blood had been centrifuged rather than merely allowed to sediment, the volume occupied by red cells may have been even less. The buffy coat is enormously increased, occupying almost two-thirds of the column of blood. This is indicative of a very high white cell count. This tube of blood can be compared with the haematocrit tubes in question 11 which have a buffy coat of normal thickness.

b. The most likely diagnosis is chronic granulocytic or chronic myeloid leukaemia. When the buffy coat is so obvious, the white cell count is usually of the order of 200–400 × 10^9/L. A striking increase of white cells, such as is seen in this specimen, gave rise to the term 'leukaemia', meaning 'white blood'.

23. The large parasite is a microfilaria, specifically *Loa loa*. In addition, there are two very small ring forms (top right) which are *Plasmodium falciparum*.

24.
a. The blood film shows poikilocytosis including the presence of target cells.

b. The presence of poikilocytosis including target cells in a patient with a normal haemoglobin concentration, a high red cell count and microcytosis suggests a diagnosis of thalassaemia trait, in this ethnic group probably beta-thalassaemia trait.

c. The diagnosis was confirmed by haemoglobin electrophoresis and documentation of an elevated haemoglobin A_2 concentration.

25. Wiskott–Aldrich syndrome is characterized by thrombocytopenia with small platelets (as can be seen from the histogram), together with eczema and immune insufficiency, the latter particularly effecting T cells and leading to recurrent infections.

26.
a. The film shows a number of irregularly contracted cells, i.e. cells which lack central pallor but are not as round and regular as spherocytes. Such cells are indicative of oxidant damage or of an unstable haemoglobin. There is also anaemia.

b. Given the history and the ethnic origin of the child, the irregularly contracted cells are likely to result from exposure to oxidant stress in a patient with deficiency of glucose-6-phosphate-dehydrogenase (G6PD). The oxidant stress could be either a drug given to treat the urinary tract infection or the effects of the infection itself.

27.
a. The films show gross elevation of the white cell count. There are increased numbers of neutrophils and the high power film

shows one eosinophil and one basophil. White cell precursors are present, specifically myelocytes, promyelocytes and blast cells.

b. The clinical and haematological features are typical of chronic granulocytic leukaemia, also referred to as chronic myeloid leukaemia.

c. This type of leukaemia is characterized by an acquired cytogenetic abnormality in the clone of neoplastic cells, specifically a translocation between chromosome 9 and chromosome 22 described as t(9;22)(q34;q11). This gives rise to a chromosome 22 with a shortened long arm which is referred to as the Philadelphia chromosome.

28.
a. The cell is a macrophage which contains *Leishmania donovani*.
b. The diagnosis is leishmaniasis.

29.
a. There is a grossly expanded buffy coat and, as the patient's white cell count is said to be normal, this is indicative of a greatly increased platelet count. The haematocrit is also increased.

b. The most likely diagnosis is a myeloproliferative disorder in which there is an increase not only in the red cell count, haemoglobin and haematocrit, but also in the platelet count. This condition is polycythaemia rubra vera. Not many patients have a platelet count increased to this extent. Had the haemoglobin and the total red cell mass been normal, the diagnosis would have been essential thrombocythaemia.

c. The patient's transient ischaemic attacks are likely to be caused by obstruction of small vessels by hyperviscous blood and by aggregated platelets.

30.
a. There is an erythematous and papular rash, and the blood film shows two abnormal lymphocytes, one of which is larger than normal, while the other shows a convoluted nucleus. This combination of features is indicative of mycosis fungoides or Sézary's syndrome.

b. Sézary's cells are of T lineage.

31.
a. The film shows numerous elliptocytes and ovalocytes. The diagnosis is hereditary elliptocytosis.

b. In the majority of patients, this disorder is of no clinical significance, not being associated with anaemia or even with significant haemolysis.

32.
a. The film shows stomatocytes and ovalocytosis. There is one macroovalocyte. This combination of features is characteristic of 'south-east Asian ovalocytosis', an inherited condition which occurs in Malaysians, Indonesians, Philippinos and the inhabitants of Papua and New Guinea and the Torres Strait

islands to the north of Queensland. An alternative name is Melanesian ovalocytosis.

b. This red cell defect is harmless in herozygotes, although epidemiological evidence suggests that the homozygous state may be incompatible with life.

33.

a. The patient is plethoric and has one gangrenous toe. The combination of these two features suggests that he has polycythaemia, possibly polycythaemia rubra vera, with vascular obstruction as a consequence of hyperviscosity. An alternative name for this condition is primary proliferative polycythaemia.

b. Useful tests are:
- full blood count, to confirm the polycythaemia and check for leucocytosis, thrombocytosis or an increased basophil count
- estimation of total red cell and plasma volume by isotopic dilution techniques to confirm that there is a true polycythaemia
- arterial oxygen saturation to exclude hypoxia as a cause of polycythaemia
- ultrasound of the abdomen to evaluate spleen size and to exclude renal cysts and tumours as a cause of polycythaemia
- bone marrow aspirate and trephine biopsy to seek evidence of a myeloproliferative disorder
- serum erythropoietin concentration to help to exclude a secondary polycythaemia.

34.

a. There are target cells, a large platelet and a cell which has points at both ends because it is partially sickled.

b. The diagnosis is compound heterozygosity for haemoglobin S and β^+-thalassaemia. The patient's genotype is S/β^+-thalassaemia. Because her β-thalassaemia gene is a β^+ gene not a β^0 gene, the patient is able to produce small amounts of normal β chain and thus small amounts of haemoglobin A. If you said the patient had sickle cell anaemia, this answer would be wrong.

c. The patient will, on average, pass on the β^s gene to half her offspring and the β^+-thalassaemia gene to half. The child has a 1 in 2 chance of inheriting a β^s gene from its father and in that case would have either sickle cell anaemia or sickle cell/β-thalassaemia compound heterozygosity.

35.

a. The blood film shows three highly abnormal lymphocytes with flower-shaped or clover leaf-shaped nuclei.

b. The most likely diagnosis is adult T-cell leukaemia/lymphoma which occurs particularly in Japanese and Afro-Caribbeans.

c. The retrovirus, HTLV-I, is an aetiological agent in this leukaemia.

d. The cranial nerve palsies are likely to be indicative of meningeal infiltration.

36.
a. The blood film shows thrombocytopenia and a giant platelet, indicating that the patient's autoimmune thrombocytopenia has recurred. Despite the history of splenectomy, there are no features of hyposplenism. The technetium scan shows isotopic uptake posteriorly in the position of the splenic bed. This indicates that the patient has a splenunculus. This may have hypertrophied and been responsible for the relapse of the thrombocytopenia.

b. The CT scan shows that the splenunculus is attached to the posterior wall of the stomach.

c. Removal of the splenunculus might lead to remission of the thrombocytopenia.

37.
a. The cells are osteoblasts. These are normal bone marrow cells which are seen more often in bone marrow aspirates from children than in those from adults.

b. Since osteoblasts are normal cells, their presence in an aspirate is not generally of any significance. However, in aspirates from adults they are usually present only in small numbers. The presence of increased numbers and clumps of osteoblasts may be indicative of bone marrow metastases with an osteoblastic reaction. Bone marrow films should therefore be examined carefully for tumour cells when large numbers of osteoblasts are seen.

38.
a. The likely diagnosis is multiple myeloma since the peripheral blood film shows rouleaux, increased background staining and the presence of a plasma cell, and the bone marrow is largely replaced by plasma cells.

b. Useful tests would be a skeletal survey, examination of the serum for a paraprotein and examination of the urine for free monoclonal light chain (Bence–Jones' protein).

c. The mechanism of the hypercalcaemia is stimulation of osteoclast activity by cytokines secreted by the myeloma cells.

39.
a. The most likely diagnosis is hereditary spherocytosis.

b. The son's film shows spherocytosis. The father's film shows spheroacanthocytes, since acanthocytosis as a consequence of splenectomy has been superimposed on spherocytosis.

40.
a. The blood film shows lymphocytosis, a smear cell and a conspicuous lack of platelets. The lymphocytes are mainly small and mature with clumped chromatin.

b. The most likely diagnosis is chronic lymphocytic leukaemia.

c. The test most useful in diagnosis would be immunophenotyping of the lymphocytes to demonstrate that they are monoclonal B cells expressing the surface membrane antigens typical of CLL.

d. The most likely cause is herpes zoster, leading to severe scarring. Note that the scar stops at the midline. Patients with chronic lymphocytic leukaemia have a greatly increased risk of herpes zoster because of their impaired cell-mediated immunity. Note that the patient has not had radiotherapy—modern radiotherapy techniques do *not* lead to scarring.

41.

a. The blood film shows five or more irregularly contracted cells. Note that, although they lack central pallor, they differ from spherocytes in having an irregular outline.

b. The Heinz body test exposes blood to a supravital dye which stains Heinz bodies. Heinz bodies are denatured haemoglobin. This Heinz body test is positive. Note that the red cell inclusions are at the periphery of the cell and sometimes protrude through the cell membrane. They are attached to the membrane by sulphydryl bonds.

c. The irregularly contracted cells and Heinz bodies are indicative of oxidant-induced haemolysis. In a patient with dermatitis herpetiformis this is likely to be due to treatment with dapsone. In a Northern European Caucasian woman, an underlying deficiency of glucose-6-phosphate dehydrogenase is quite unlikely.

42.

Blood film (A) shows platelet satellitism—the platelet count would be invalid because platelets which are adherent to a white cell will pass through the counting chamber of automated counters with the white cell and will not be recognized as platelets.

(B) Shows platelet aggregation—the masses of platelets are too large to be recognized as platelets; individual platelets within the masses will not be recognized and counted so the count will be invalid.

(C) Shows fibrin strands—this phenomenon indicates that coagulation is occurring within the blood sample, either because of a hypercoagulable state in the patient or because there has been difficulty with venepuncture; platelets will also be consumed in this process and the count is likely to be invalid.

(D) Shows thrombocytopenia—this film shows a marked reduction of platelets and no abnormality, which would suggest a factitious result; it is likely that the platelet count is valid.

43.
a. The film shows numerous platelets, 'packed' red cells, two neutrophils and two basophils, suggesting that the haemoglobin concentration, white cell count, basophil count and platelet count are all elevated.
b. The most likely diagnosis is polycythaemia rubra vera.
c. The patient's back shows scratch marks, indicating that he is suffering from pruritus. This is likely to be caused by the release of histamine from the numerous basophils. Patients often notice that the itch is worse after a hot bath.

44.
a. There is increased rouleaux formation and two atypical lymphocytes. One of these is very large with an immature chromatin pattern and cytoplasmic basophilia, particularly at the periphery of the cell.
b. The most likely diagnosis is infectious mononucleosis or glandular fever.
c. A screening test for the Paul–Bunnell antibody is indicated.

45.
a. There is neutrophil leucocytosis with toxic granulation.
b. These changes are non-specific but would support a diagnosis of bacterial pneumonia.

46.
The stain in (A) is positive for iron and indicates that the patient has normal iron stores (within the bone marrow macrophages).

The stain in (B) is negative for iron and indicates absent iron stores. A significant proportion of healthy women in the reproductive age range have absent iron stores, but if the patient is anaemic the absence of iron stores would support a diagnosis of iron deficiency anaemia.

47.
a. The trephine biopsy shows infiltration of the bone marrow by adenocarcinoma. Acinus formation is apparent.
b. The likely diagnosis is metastatic carcinoma of the prostate.

48.
a. There has been necrosis and sloughing of the skin.
b. The abnormality suggests that there has been extravasation of a highly irritant drug such as doxorubicin.

49.
a. The serum shows precipitation of a cryoglobulin while the blood film shows that a leucocyte, probably a monocyte, has phagocytosed globules of cryoglobulin.
b. Multiple myeloma or Waldenström's macroglobulinaemia could provide an explanation.

50.
The film shows a binucleated Gaucher's cell. The diagnosis is Gaucher's disease.

51.
a. The principle of the test is that acidification of the blood leads to normal red cells being lysed while fetal red cells (or other cells containing haemoglobin F) remain intact.

b. This film shows a neutrophil, an intact fetal red cell and the ghosts of maternal red cell. The presence of a fetal red cell indicates that a feto-maternal haemorrhage has occurred.

52.
a. The radiographs show progressive destruction and collapse of vertebrae.
b. The most likely diagnosis is multiple myeloma.

53.
a. The vertebra shows myelomatous deposits.
b. The sternum has been split down the centre to show myelomatous deposits; there has also been a pathological fracture with subsequent misalignment of the top and bottom parts of the sternum.

54.
The patient's three neutrophils show no alkaline phosphatase activity at all. A low neutrophil alkaline phosphatase score favours a diagnosis of chronic granulocytic leukaemia since it is low in about 95% of patients.

55.
a. The throat shows marked tonsillar enlargement and superficial white areas which are likely to represent necrotic tissue and leucocytes that are part of the inflammatory response.
b. The trunk shows a macular rash.
c. In view of the blood count and blood film findings, these abnormalities are most likely to be caused by infectious mononucleosis.
d. This condition is caused by primary infection by the Epstein-Barr virus (EBV).

56.
a. The film shows rather pleomorphic blast cells, anaemia and thrombocytopenia.
b. The chest X-ray shows gross mediastinal widening, suggestive of gross thymic enlargement.
c. The likely diagnosis is acute lymphoblastic leukaemia.
d. In view of the thymic enlargement, it is likely that this is of T lineage.

57.
a. Pleomorphic plasma cells including plasmablasts are apparent. Note that some have a clock-face chromatic pattern, an eccentric nucleus and a Golgi zone, permitting the lineage to be recognized. Others are more abnormal and not so easily recognized.
b. The plasma cells show a positive reaction for lambda light chain and a negative reaction for kappa light chain, i.e. they are monoclonal.
c. The diagnosis is multiple myeloma.

58.
a. The blood film shows at least three red cell fragments or schistocytes.

b. Urinary haemosiderin is present, being responsible for the large amounts of material staining blue-black with a stain for iron.

c. These findings are indicative of a mechanical haemolytic anaemia.

59. The most likely diagnosis is haemophilia.

60.
a. The bone marrow film shows grossly abnormal multinucleated erythroblasts. In addition, two myeloblasts are present.

b. The most likely diagnosis is acute myeloid leukaemia of M6 type, otherwise known as erythroleukaemia.

61.
a. The bone marrow aspirate shows hypergranular promyelocytes, one of which (centre) has a giant granule.

b. The coagulation tests show that the patient has disseminated intravascular coagulation ('DIC').

c. The diagnosis is acute hypergranular promyelocytic leukaemia or acute myeloid leukaemia, type M3.

d. The cytogenetic abnormality expected is t(15;17)(q22;q21).

62.
a. There is acanthocytosis and macrocytosis.

b. Acanthocytosis in liver disease (also called 'spur cell haemolytic anaemia') is of grave prognostic significance.

63.
a. In addition to the hysterectomy scar, the abdomen shows pigmentation due to application of heat, known as 'erythema ab igneum'.

b. In view of the patient's history, she has probably been putting a hot water bottle on the abdomen in an attempt to relieve severe pain caused by recurrence of her Hodgkin's disease.

64.
a. The blood film shows target cells and two irregularly contracted cells.

b. The electrophoretic strip shows two bands, one with the mobility of haemoglobin A and the other with the mobility of haemoglobin C or E. Since the patient is Afro-Caribbean, the abnormal haemoglobin is much more likely to be haemoglobin C than haemoglobin E and the diagnosis is haemoglobin C trait.

65. Both the aspirate and the trephine biopsy show fungi, specifically *Cryptococcus neoformans*. The patient has cryptococcosis, which is one of the opportunistic infections that occur in AIDS.

66.

a. The blood film shows two lymphocytes and a monocyte. One of the lymphocytes has a deeply cleft nucleus and the other is very small with very scanty cytoplasm. The trephine biopsy shows a paratrabecular lymphoid infiltrate. The lymph node biopsy shows effacement of the lymph node by a lymphoma with a follicular growth pattern. There is infiltration of the perinodal fat.

b. The diagnosis is follicular lymphoma. The cytological features of the circulating lymphoma cells, the pattern of bone marrow infiltration and the follicular growth pattern in the lymph node are all typical of this lymphoma.

67.

a. There is increased rouleaux formation. The two white cells are a neutrophil and a granular lymphocyte. The likely causes are (1) an increase in polyclonal immunoglobulins, (2) the presence of a monoclonal immunoglobulin, or (3) an increased concentration of 'acute phase reactants' such as fibrinogen and α_2 macroglobulin. This particular patient had a monoclonal immunoglobulin, i.e. a paraprotein, and light-chain associated amyloidosis.

b. There are red cell agglutinates. This is indicative of a cold agglutinin, i.e. a red cell agglutinin which is active at low temperatures. Underlying causes include infections, such as mycoplasma infection or infectious mononucleosis, and lymphoproliferative disorders.

68.

a. The red cell cytogram shows a second population of cells above the normal red cell cluster. These are red cell agglutinates, which are larger than single red cells and lead to a factitious macrocytosis.

b. The presence of red cell agglutinates is likely to indicate the presence of cold agglutinins since warm antibodies do not cause agglutination of red cells at normal laboratory temperatures.

69.

Curve A shows decreased osmotic fragility. The final diagnosis was pyruvate kinase deficiency, the commonest of the congenital non-spherocytic haemolytic anaemias.

Curve B shows markedly increased osmotic fragility. The final diagnosis was hereditary spherocytosis. It should be noted that any other anaemia with large numbers of spherocytes, e.g. autoimmune haemolytic anaemia, would have a similar osmotic fragility curve.

70.

a. The film does not show any sickle cells but shows small dense deformed cells. These are described as irregularly contracted cells. In this case, they appear to contain straight-edged crystals. This indicates the presence of haemoglobin C.

b. Since the patient has both a positive sickle solubility test and red cells, suggesting the presence of haemoglobin C, the likely diagnosis is compound heterozygosity for haemoglobins S and C. The genotype, instead of being $\beta\beta$, is $\beta^s\beta^c$. The patient has no normal β genes and so cannot synthesize haemoglobin A.

c. Sickle cell/haemoglobin C disease causes a clinical disorder similar to sickle cell anaemia although it is, on average, somewhat less severe.

71.
a. The skin biopsy shows a lymphoid infiltrate in the upper dermis and within the epidermis, infiltrates of the latter type being referred to as Pautrier's microabscesses. The electron micrograph shows a highly complex or 'convoluted' nucleus.

b. The diagnosis is mycosis fungoides or, since there are abnormal circulating lymphocytes, Sézary's syndrome. These are two aspects of the one disease, both included under the umbrella term of cutaneous T cell lymphoma.

72.
a. There is considerable abdominal enlargement. Possible causes would include hepatosplenomegaly and ascites. The CT scan shows very marked splenic enlargement.

b. Pancytopenia, a leucoerythroblastic blood film and gross splenomegaly suggest a diagnosis of idiopathic myelofibrosis, also referred to as myelofibrosis with myeloid metaplasia.

73. The diagnosis is Burkitt's lymphoma or acute lymphoblastic leukaemia of L3 type. Note the cytoplasmic basophilia and vacuolation of the lymphoblasts and the 'starry sky' appearance of the lymph node biopsy. The starry sky appearance is caused by the presence of macrophages within the lymphomatous tissue as a consequence of a very high rate of cell turnover and death.

74. There are large lymphoid cells with prominent nucleoli. The nuclei have some chromatin condensation and hence are not lymphoblasts. The diagnosis was prolymphocytic leukaemia of B lineage.

75.
a. Patient b has a small discrete band in the γ globulin region and reduction of normal immunoglobulins.

b. Patient c has a heavy band in the β globulin region and a reduction of normal immunoglobulins. These are monoclonal immunoglobulins or paraproteins.

c. Both patients had multiple myeloma.

76.
a. Patient 1 has a positive sickle solubility test and both haemoglobin A and haemoglobin S. The diagnosis is sickle cell trait. A positive sickle solubility test produces turbidity so that lines printed on a piece of cardboard cannot be seen clearly through the turbid lysate.
b. Patient 2 has haemoglobin A and an abnormal band with the same mobility as haemoglobin S. However, the sickle solubility test is negative. This is likely to represent the heterozygous state for one of the non-sickling haemoglobins referred to as haemoglobin D or haemoglobin G. In this patient, the diagnosis was heterozygosity for haemoglobin D Punjab.

77.
a. The diagnosis is nodular sclerosing Hodgkin's disease. Note the bands of collagen, the two or three binucleated Reed–Sternberg cells and the mononuclear Hodgkin's cells.
b. The largest cell is a Reed–Sternberg cell. Note that it is a very large and binucleate cell. The nuclei both contain giant nucleoli. There is a somewhat smaller bare nucleus with a large central nucleolus. This is the nucleus of a mononuclear Hodgkin's cell. The Reed–Sternberg cells and the Hodgkin's cells are the neoplastic cells in this disease. The more numerous lymphocytes are reactive.

78.
a. The urine does not contain a paraprotein but contains traces of normal serum globulins. This is indicative of renal damage.
b. The urine contains normal serum proteins and a discrete homogeneous band moving between the β and γ globulins. This is a monoclonal light chain band, also known as a Bence–Jones protein. The presence of normal serum globulins is again indicative of renal damage.
c. The urine contains albumin and a discrete abnormal band with α_2 mobility which is a Bence–Jones protein.

79.
a. The blood film shows anisocytosis and poikilocytosis, including elliptocytes and a tear drop poikilocyte. There is a minor population of hypochromic microcytes, rendering the film dimorphic.
b. There are four erythroblasts. One of these shows very defective cytoplasmic haemoglobinization; this is the explanation of the hypochromic microcytes in the blood.
c. The iron stains show increased storage iron and the presence of ring sideroblasts.
d. In this patient, this was an acquired disorder, one of the myelodysplastic syndromes, referred to as refractory anaemia with ring sideroblasts or primary acquired sideroblastic anaemia.

80.
a. There is gum hyperplasia. The bone marrow photograph shows five very large blast cells with abundant cytoplasm and prominent nucleoli; these are monoblasts.
b. The diagnosis is acute monoblastic leukaemia. Gum infiltration is typical of acute leukaemia with a monocytic component.

81.
a. The May–Grünwald–Giemsa stain shows four very abnormal cells which do not resemble any known haemopoietic cells. The cytokeratin stain is positive, indicating that these are of epithelial origin.
b. The diagnosis is metastatic carcinoma, in this case from a primary carcinoma of the breast.

82.
a. There is gross enlargement of para-aortic lymph nodes.
b. The most likely diagnosis is lymphoma, in this case Hodgkin's disease. A metastatic tumour, e.g. germ cell tumour of the testis, is also a possibility.

83.
a. The bone marrow shows three very large cells which are megakaryocytes.
b. This indicates that the thrombocytopenia is not likely to be due to reduction of megakaryocyte numbers and supports a diagnosis of autoimmune thrombocytopenic purpura.

84.
a. The patient's arm shows linear petechiae.
b. This could indicate either a factitious (i.e. deliberately self-induced) lesion or severe thrombocytopenia with a light scratch having led to this distribution of petechiae. In this patient, the latter explanation was correct.

85.
These implements are used for measuring the bleeding time. One is a lancet and the others are devices for measuring a template bleeding time in which an incision of defined length and depth is made.

86.
The vascular abnormalities of the lips indicate that the patient has hereditary haemorrhagic telangiectasia. This condition has an autosomal dominant inheritance. Presentation is usually with epistaxis. Gastrointestinal bleeding from vascular lesions in the intestine is also common.

87.
a. There is virtually no aggregation with ADP (adenosine diphosphate) and adrenaline, while aggregation with ristocetin is reduced.
b. The history and the almost absent platelet aggregation indicate a severe inherited defect of platelet function, in this case with normal-sized platelets and a normal platelet count.

The diagnosis was thrombasthenia (Glanzmann's thrombasthenia).

88.
a. There is marked cervical lymphadenopathy in both the anterior and posterior triangles.
b. There is an unusually severe reaction to a smallpox vaccination.
c. Both patients had chronic lymphocytic leukaemia. When smallpox vaccination was practised, such patients often developed large local lesions and sometimes disseminated vaccinia after vaccination, an indication of the impaired T cell function in this type of leukaemia.

89.
a. The film show a nucleated red cell (normoblast) and a myelocyte. There is therefore a leucoerythroblastic blood film, and tear drop poikilocytes are also present. The bone marrow shows replacement of haemopoietic tissue by fibroblasts and collagen. Reticulin is greatly increased with parallel strands.
b. The diagnosis is idiopathic myelofibrosis. This is a myeloproliferative disorder in which the fibrosis is reactive to a proliferation of abnormal haematopoietic cells.

90.
a. Lytic lesions of multiple myeloma.
b. Lytic lesions of multiple myeloma plus greatly thickened bone of Paget's disease.

91.
a. The blood film shows microcytosis, target cells and marked poikilocytosis. The blood count show anaemia, microcytosis, reduced MCH and MCHC and increased RDW (red cell distribution width, indicative of anisocytosis).
b. The red cell cytogram shows markedly hypochromic and microcytic cells, reflected in the low MCHC and MCV. The RDW is greatly increased, reflecting anisocytosis. The increased HDW (haemoglobin distribution width) reflects anisochromasia, i.e. variation of haemoglobin concentration from cell to cell.
c. The diagnosis was haemoglobin H disease. The abnormalities in the film and the blood count are too marked to be suggestive of β-thalassaemia trait.

92.
a. The chest X-ray shows a mass in the position of the thymus. In a patient with pure red cell aplasia, this is likely to be a thymoma.
b. The pure red cell aplasia is autoimmune in origin.

93.
a. The thrombocythaemia is not well controlled. The platelet count is obviously still very high.

b. There is anisocytosis and poikilocytosis and two severely hypochromic cells, making the film dimorphic. One of the hypochromic cells (on the edge of the film) contains a Pappenheimer body.

c. The patient is anaemic and the blood film suggests that the patient probably has a sideroblastic anaemia. This is indicative of myelodysplasia, either as part of the natural history of the disease or as a long-term consequence of the ^{32}P therapy. Myelodysplastic changes in patients with myeloproliferative disorders may precede the development of acute leukaemia.

94. Positive reactions are shown by agglutinated cells which sink to the bottom of the well and form a compact clump. Non-agglutinated cells remain dispersed. Note that all the saline controls are negative.

a. Patient 1 is AB positive; his cells are agglutinated by anti-A, anti-B, anti-A+B and anti-D; his serum does not agglutinate either A or B cells.

b. Patient 2 is O negative; his red cells are not agglutinated by any of the antisera while his serum contains anti-A and anti-B.

c. Patient 3 is B positive; his cells are agglutinated by anti-B, anti-A+B and anti-D but not anti-A, while his serum contains anti-A but not anti-B.

95. a. There are three or four spherocytes.

b. It is likely that the baby has ABO haemolytic disease of the newborn, caused by maternal anti-A crossing the placenta and damaging fetal red cells. Hereditary spherocytosis is also possible.

96. a. The skull shows a 'hair-on-end' appearance consistent with marked expansion of haemopoietic bone marrow. The clinical photograph shows an ulcer on the ankle of a patient who appears to be African or Afro-Caribbean.

b. This combination of abnormalities suggests sickle cell anaemia.

97. a. Angular cheilosis.

b. Koilonychia.

c. Iron deficiency.

98. There are haemorrhagic bullae on mucous membranes. The likely cause is very severe thrombocytopenia, either autoimmune in origin or due to an immunological reaction to a drug, with platelets being damaged by an innocent bystander mechanism.

99.
a. Eosinophils.
b. Causes include allergy (e.g. asthma, hay fever, drug allergy), parasites (e.g. hookworm), skin diseases (e.g. pemphigus), eosinophilic leukaemia and the therapeutic use of growth factors. Sometimes the cause of eosinophilia cannot be determined (idiopathic eosinophilia). In this patient, the cause was administration of interleukin 3.

100.
a. The photograph shows a blast cell (centre) and two neutrophils with reduced nuclear lobulation. The latter is referred to as an acquired Pelger–Hüet anomaly. In addition, the red cells show anisocytosis and poikilocytosis.
b. These findings are indicative of either a myelodysplastic syndrome (MDS) or acute myeloid leukaemia (AML) which has occurred as part of the natural history of polycythaemia rubra vera or as a consequence of the ^{32}P therapy. A bone marrow examination to determine the number of blasts would be necessary to distinguish between MDS and AML. This patient had between 20 and 30% bone marrow blasts and the condition was therefore categorized as refractory anaemia with excess of blasts in transformation (RAEB-T), one of the myelodysplastic syndromes.

101.
a. There is swelling of the knee and, in addition, the calf muscles appear wasted. In view of the family history, it is likely that the patient has a haemarthrosis as a consequence of haemophilia. The wasting of the calf muscles has resulted from immobilization during previous haemarthroses.
b. Such manifestations of haemophilia are much less common nowadays because the ready availability of factor VIII concentrates permits early and more effective treatment of bleeding episodes.

102.
a. The cell is a lymphocyte showing heavy cytoplasmic vacuolation.
b. This abnormality is usually consequent on an inborn error of metabolism. In this case, the child had I cell disease. Other causes of vacuolated lymphocytes include the mucopolysaccharidoses, Niemann–Pick disease, Wolman's disease, Pompey's disease, Tay–Sach's disease, Batten–Spielmeyer–Vogt disease and Jordan's anomaly.

103.
a. There are two neutrophils with reduced lobulation, one of which has a shape resembling that of peanut and the other resembling a pair of spectacles. This abnormality is indicative of the Pelger–Hüet anomaly, an inherited condition with an autosomal dominant inheritance.
b. This anomaly has no clinical significance, unlike the acquired

Pelger–Hüet anomaly which is indicative of a myelodysplastic syndrome (MDS). In the acquired condition, the blood count is likely to be abnormal and the peripheral blood and bone marrow films usually show other abnormalities indicative of MDS.

104.
a. The lymphocyte shows a large pink-staining granule and the neutrophil shows giant granules with anomalous staining characteristics.
b. These abnormalities are indicative of the Chédiak–Higashi syndrome. This is a serious inherited disorder with an autosomal recessive inheritance characterized by partial oculocutaneous albinism, neurological abnormalities, susceptibility to infection and, ultimately, hepatosplenomegaly and pancytopenia consequent on proliferation of haemophagocytic histiocytes.

105.
a. The acid lysis test is a test for the susceptibility of red cells to lysis on exposure to acidified serum containing complement. The test illustrated is positive as there is lysis of the patient's red cells only in fresh acidified serum. The test is negative when serum is not acidified and when complement in the serum has been inactivated by exposure to heat.
b. The patient's history is suggestive of paroxysmal nocturnal haemoglobinuria (PNH). This diagnosis is confirmed by the positive acid lysis test, also known as a Ham's test.

106.
a. There is a short, mispositioned thumb. Radiology showed hypoplasia of the metacarpal.
b. The diagnosis is Fanconi's anaemia. This is a congenital disorder with an autosomal recessive inheritance, usually leading to the onset of cytopenia during childhood or adolescence. Other abnormalities are common, particularly growth retardation, microthalmia and abnormalities of the thumbs and radii.

107.
a. There is radial deviation of the wrist, indicative of an absent radius.
b. This is a syndrome known as thrombocytopenia with absent radius (TAR) syndrome. Inheritance is autosomal recessive. It is characterized by bilateral absence of the radii and severe thrombocytopenia, present at birth, with very marked reduction of bone marrow megakaryocytes.

108.
a. The blood film shows thrombocytopenia, giant platelets and a cytoplasmic inclusion in the neutrophil which resembles a Döhle body.
b. This combination of abnormalities is indicative of the

May–Hegglin anomaly, a congenital disorder with an autosomal dominant inheritance. This condition may be asymptomatic or may cause a bleeding tendency of mild or moderate severity, depending on the severity of the thrombocytopenia.

109.

a. These are pigment stones, reflecting increased breakdown of haemoglobin.

b. Any very chronic haemolytic anaemia may lead to the formation of pigment gallstones. Pigment stones are very common in sickle cell anaemia and may also be seen in other haemoglobinopathies and in inherited defects of the red cell membrane such as hereditary spherocytosis. This particular patient had haemoglobin C disease.

Further Reading

Bain BJ 1995 Blood cells, 2nd edn. Blackwell Science, Oxford

Bain BJ 1996 Beginners' guide to blood cells. Blackwell Science, Oxford

Bain BJ 1998 Self-assessment for the MRCP: haematology. Imperial College Press, London

Linch DC, Yates AP, Watts MJ 1996 Colour guide: haematology. Churchill Livingstone, Edinburgh

Smith H 1996 Diagnosis in paediatric haematology. Churchill Livingstone, Edinburgh

Wickramasinghe SN (ed.) 1986 Systemic pathology, 3rd edn. Blood and bone marrow. Churchill Livingstone, Edinburgh, vol 2

Index

NB: entries are indexed **by question and answer numbers**.